THE LONGEVITY EQUATION

HOW TO EAT AS MUCH AS YOU LIKE AND STILL LIVE OVER 100 YEARS TO TELL ABOUT IT!

Richard G. Deeb

Illustrations by Warren Burker
Recipes by Beth Burker

LONG LIFE PRESS
Port Richey, Florida

Library of Congress Catalog Card Number: 92-90496

ISBN 0-9634020-0-5

Printed in the United States of America

Long Life Press
6709 Ridge Rd., Suite 300
Port Richey, Florida 34668

First Edition

To the memory of my father, Richard J. Deeb.
For the love, courage and wisdom he showed
me throughout my life.

ACKNOWLEDGEMENTS

I wish to express my deep appreciation and gratitude to my family and friends for all their support.

Beth and Warren Burker for the wonderful recipes and delightful illustrations.

Kathleen Lange for her insightful editing and good advice.

A Note to the Reader

CONTENTS

Foreword 13

Introduction 15

Chapter 1 Human Lifespan 19

How Long Are We Really Supposed to Live?
Why Do We No Longer Live To Our Biological Potential?

Chapter 2 The Diet for Maximum Protection 28

The Choice Foods
Protein: How Much do You Need?
Vegetarianism
Combinations for Maximum Nutrient Balance
Food Preparation
The Importance of Water
Low-Protein Food Choices
Low-Fat Food Choices
High-Complex Carbohydrates
Re-Evaluating Food

Chapter 3 Exercise 41

What Part Does it Play in the Equation?
Aerobics
Resistance/Strengthening Exercises
Flexibility

Stress-Reduction Exercises
Rehabilitative Exercises
Diet for Maximum Performance

Chapter 4 Weight Loss Strategies 74

Popular Weight-Loss Programs
Calorie-Restricted Diets
High-Protein Diets
The Lifetime Diet
Calories Don't Count
Low Protein is the Way to Go
Fat Should be 10-15% of Your Calories
High-Complex Carbohydrates are the Answer
The Lifetime Diet Summary

Chapter 5 Heart Disease 88

What is Heart Disease?
High Blood Pressure and Sodium
The Infamous Cholesterol Connection
What is the Main Cause of Heart Disease?
What Can We Do to Prevent It?
What Can We Do to Reverse It?

Chapter 6 Cancer 121

What is Cancer?
Initiation and Promotion
The Secret is to Prevent
Antioxidants and Cancer
Fiber and Cancer
Exercise and Cancer
New on the Horizon: Designer Foods

Chapter 7 Osteoporosis 140

How Serious of a Threat is Osteoporosis?
What Are Bones Anyway?
Exercise and Osteoporosis
The Main Cause of Osteoporosis
High Dairy Consumption is Not the Answer

Chapter 8 Diabetes 152

What is Diabetes?
Traditional Approach to Diabetes
Better Strategies for Controlling Diabetes

Chapter 9 In the Balance 159

The Lifetime Diet Guide 164

Fast Food Tables 166
Smart Food Tables 176
12 - Day Food Plan 181
Healthful Recipes 194
Food Value Tables 225

Index of Tables and Charts 235

Notes 236

Bibliography 241

FOREWORD

Some people leave indelible impressions in your mind. Ethel Morton is one of those people for me. Her strength of character, intelligence, and positive attitude stand out above the crowd. She is living proof for the validity of this book.

"I've never had fried food in my entire life," she told me one day when I was talking to her about my Lifetime Diet Plan.

The most notable thing about this statement is that Ethel's "entire life" has thus far involved nearly 100 years - and she is still in remarkably good physical, mental and spiritual condition. As I looked into her alert, intelligent eyes and noted her strong, slender build and clear skin, I thought, "Yes, the proof's definitely shown up in the pudding here."

Ethel has always been a vegetarian, even before vegetarianism became popular. She has been an example of what a careful diet and a balanced way of life can do. She attributes her health and vigor at the age of 99 to a combination of her vegetarian diet, proper exercise, lots of water, continual education of the mind, and a positive attitude. And she has two masters degrees, a Ph.D., a strong posture, and a healthy radiance to show for it.

"A positive mental attitude is essential to keep you healthy and strong," Ethel insists. "Each of us comes into the world with a talent. If we don't use it, we lose it. Never think, 'I can't.' You never accomplish anything until you try. Look for inspiration, then make a positive plan. An idea may come from God, but you need to do something in response to it. Imagination has a great deal to do with your success. Visualize yourself as succeeding. Be sure of what you want, believe in it, and pursue it."

If you choose to look at the bright side of life, you will not only improve the quality of your life, but may very likely increase the length of it. If we could choose a long life without happiness, would we want it? Still, most of us reach for it, even without it's guarantees. Perhaps we're all a people of hope. "Without a vision, the people perish," the Scriptures say. So we go on searching for that ultimate Fountain of Youth, assuming that with such youth comes hope of joy. With health of body, soul, and spirit, long life becomes very desirable.

Ethel has been an ongoing inspiration to me while writing this book, and will continue to inspire me as I live out the Lifetime Plan she exemplifies.

INTRODUCTION

Many people in my business and family circle have asked me for nutritional advice over the years, knowing I had spent years of research on the subject. So I started to compile my notes as a reference manual to aid quick retrieval of my research when needed. Then friends started to ask me for copies of my notes. One thing led to another, until finally I thought, "Why not write a book and let the whole public in on it?"

The main thing I want to "let you in on" in this book is that you don't have to settle for a life span of 78 years "if you're lucky." We humans are designed to live 120 years. Anything less than that should be termed as premature death. In the following chapters, I describe the factors which cause this premature death and how we can, with lifestyle changes, prevent them and live up to our biological potential of 120 years or even longer!

Although there is no simple equation for longevity, there are some key principles we can apply to our lifestyles which can potentially increase our life spans to well over 100 years. While it's true that proper diet and exercise alone will not necessarily lead to a long, healthy life, these two elements are key ingredients to the recipe for "longevity." Out of the many other ingredients necessary (some of which I will touch upon in Chapter 1) to achieve a longer, more fulfilling life, I have elected to focus on these two key ingredients.

In my personal quest for supreme health, I have seen countless theories and quick-fix diet fads come and go. One thing I have learned is that there are no quick-fix solutions to supreme health. There are only carefully planned, lifelong programs based on already existing, scientifically-proven human and animal studies.

I have read and studied countless books and research articles by medical and nutritional health care professionals which have contributed to some helpful findings regarding longevity guidelines. The evidence is startling and exciting! The news I now share in this book does not involve any "golden fleeces" or new wonder drugs, but introduces a *total way of life* which is not only longer, but stronger, healthier and more enjoyable.

HERE'S TO YOU

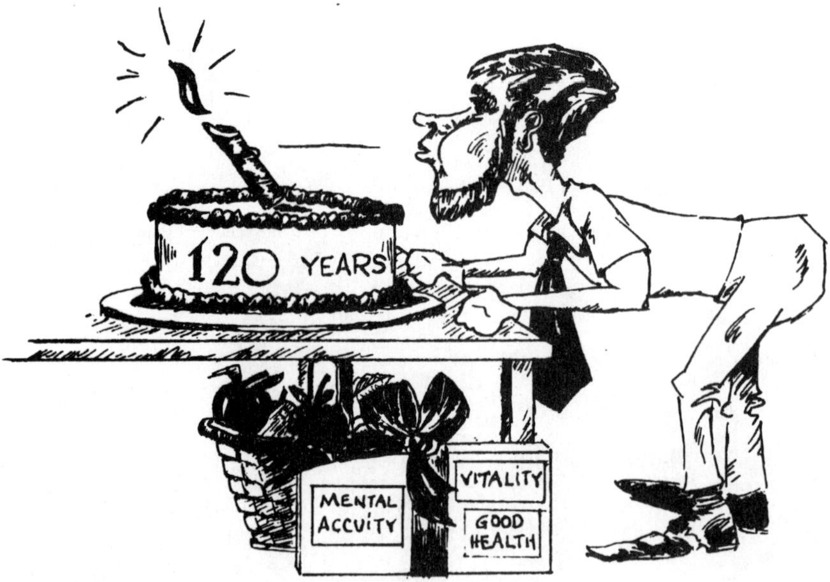

AND YOUR 120th BIRTHDAY CELEBRATION!

Chapter 1

HUMAN LIFESPAN

How Long Are We Really Supposed to Live?

THIS is a question many a person has pondered. Over the centuries, the quest for the answer to this question has, at times, been at a feverish pace. Writers, scientists, artists, philosophers, and physicians have all sought for the magical "Fountain of Youth."

Many longevity experts today peg the maximum human life span at approximately 120 years. This ties in with the Biblical reference in the Book of Genesis which indicates that man is designed to live 120 years. For though "he is indeed flesh; yet his days shall be one hundred and twenty years." [Gen. 6:3]

The Bible tells us that we can increase our longevity by following certain guidelines. Some of these guidelines are spiritual in nature [ie, if we honor our parents, we are told we will increase our years and bring a blessing into our lives (Ex. 20:12; Eph. 6:2-3); and, if we obey the commands of God, we are promised a fuller, more abundant life (Proverbs 3:1-2; 4:10; 9:10-11; Psalms 91:9-10, 15-16; John 10:10; etc.)]. Others are practical and physical (ie, rules about which foods to eat, which foods to avoid, how to prepare them, what food combinations to use or avoid, instructions regarding hygiene, sanitation, diseases, exercise, diet, etc.).

People who lived during Biblical times tended to get more "hearty" (excuse the pun) exercise, more natural foods and herbs, and, if they obeyed the Jewish laws regarding hygiene, food combinations, diet and exercise, more vigorous lives resulted.

If we were to delve into the history of varying durations of human life spans, we would begin to see patterns of shortened and lengthened averages according to how closely these Biblical guidelines were followed. The average human life expectancy during the Middle Ages, for instance, was much shorter than it is today due to poor diet, poor public sanitation, poor personal hygiene, faulty exercise habits, and a general carelessness in lifestyle.

In the past two decades, Americans have taken a renewed interest in health and fitness. If the trend continues to move toward the more "natural" lifestyle we were designed for, we may very well see an increase in longevity. Unfortunately, however, we Americans are currently bombarded with a barrage of conflicting opinions about proper diet, exercise and health care. Even the experts haven't got it all sorted out yet, so how are the rest of us to make a decision?

While it's true that different individuals will have different needs in diet, exercise, and life habits, we could also have avoided many of these specialized individual needs (which are often brought on by wrong health habits during either prenatal years, early childhood, or early adulthood) had we all followed the "correct guidelines" from the start.

Unfortunately, there is no one quick recipe for longevity. Longevity is the result of a number of factors applied throughout an individual's life. No one can guarantee a long, full life for anyone, even if all the "right rules" are followed. But why should we continue to shortcut ourselves more than necessary? The "average" life expectancy rate should not have to be less than what we were designed for.

The ideal goal to achieve a longer, more fulfilling life is of course to incorporate a ***balance*** of proper diet, rest, water intake, and spiritual, mental, physical and emotional conditioning (which includes exercise and nutrition). To focus on only one aspect of our existence (such as diet alone) is to miss the point. Since all of us are made up of body, soul and spirit, we need to take care of each part in balance. To neglect the body is to ultimately cause distress to our soul (mind/emotions) and spirit (personality/character/morals). Likewise, the mistreating of our soul or spirit will eventually take its toll on our body. (If, for instance, you eat the healthiest of foods, do all the right exercises, and do everything in your power to take proper care of your body, but then you lead a promiscuous lifestyle, you are risking any number of sexually transmitted diseases, which could ultimately destroy the very body you have tried so hard to nurture.) Each aspect of our being is so closely interwoven that our treatment (whether good or bad) of each part affects the whole.

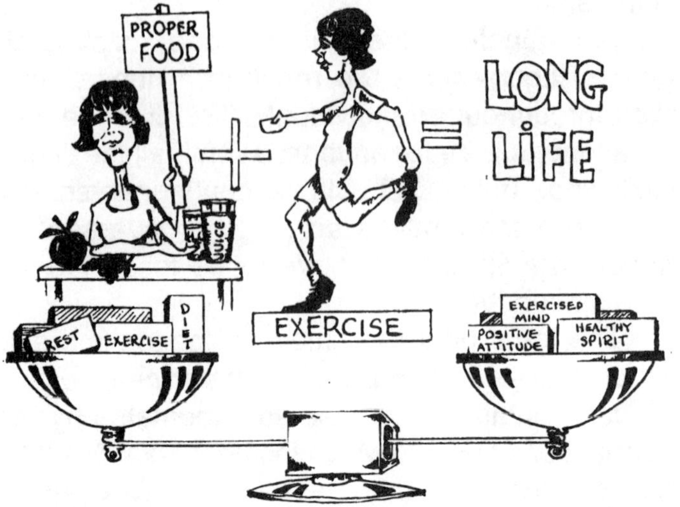

Living Proof

Throughout recorded history, many accounts of long-lived people have been documented. Such people have not only lived long, but have also led active, productive lives. Michelangelo of the Italian Renaissance era remained the architect in charge of building St. Peter's Cathedral in Rome until his death at the age of 89. George Bernard Shaw wrote *Farfetched Fables* at the age of 93. George Abbott, a Broadway actor, writer, and producer, was still directing at 100 years old.

And then there's my friend, Ethel.

Ethel's Story

Ethel Morton was born in rural England in the late 1890s. She knew kings and queens of England whom you and I could only know through history books of times long past. She's quite a remarkable woman.

Early in life, Ethel's mother decided that her family was going to live on a vegetarian diet. This type of diet was considered a fad diet at the time. Her mother was convinced, however, that this approach to eating was the way humans were intended to eat. Friends and relatives looked on her with scorn for making such a decision, saying that a person couldn't survive long on such a diet.

Through the years, Ethel has found her diet and lifestyle to be of great benefit during the trials and tribulations that life has seen fit to throw her way. She has thrived well into her late nineties on a low-fat, high-complex carbohydrate, vegetarian diet. Her husband of seventy years also did well on the same diet, until his death at 94 years of age.

Ethel relates that, in addition to a proper diet, exercise of the body and mind are keys to longevity. She tells of how she and her husband would walk several miles a day through Central Park in beautiful New York City in the 1930s and 1940s. She also believes in continual education of the mind as a way of staying forever young. She backed that up with action by receiving a doctoral degree. Even today, she still attempts to learn something new whenever possible.

I believe Ethel holds the keys to health and longevity. Her presence of mind and remarkably healthy body and spirit are a testament to her way of life. My family and friends are looking forward to a grand celebration with her next year on her 100th birthday. We could all learn a thing or two from Ethel.

The Importance of Diet and Exercise

There are several factors common among the long-lived people of the world. These factors undoubtedly contribute to their long lives. *Diet* is one of the most important factors in their longevity. The diet of long-lived people consists mainly of vegetarian, low-fat, low-calorie foods.

The Vilcabamba natives of South America are a primitive rural society. Their lifestyle includes vigorous outdoor activities and simple unrefined diets. Studies performed on the Vilcabambas indicate that they are almost entirely free of artery disease. These villagers eat mainly vegetarian foods made up of half the protein and one-third the calories of the average American diet.[1]

Another common factor in long-lived people is a history of *physical activity*. The Vilcabambas' and other long-lived communities make vigorous physical activity a part of their daily way of life. The types of physical activity involve walking, hill climbing, and vigorous outdoor work *daily*, as opposed to a half-hour aerobics class three times a week.

One example of an American who lives this type of lifestyle is Jack LaLanne. Some of us may remember Jack LaLanne's daily fitness program on television. Jack's program was the first TV Fitness Show to praise the effects of aerobic fitness -- long before aerobic fitness became popular. Jack LaLanne always celebrated his age. He was neither afraid nor hindered by it. On his 70th birthday, he swam 1-1/2 miles in Long Beach Harbor, New York, handcuffed and shackled, towing 70 boats which carried friends and reporters the entire distance! [2]

Jack LaLanne's vigorous approach to life should be a shining example of what is possible for the rest of us. People are beginning to get the message. They are beginning to understand how diet, exercise, and lifestyle affect longevity. The Bureau of Census recently projected that, by the year 2000, there will be approximately 100,000 people aged 100 years or older. The Bureau also predicts that by the year 2050 there will be about one million people living to the age of 100. Significant documented proof indicates that many humans have lived to more than one hundred years old -- evidence which suggests that the maximum human life span is well above the 100-year mark!

Why Do We No Longer Live To Our Biological Potential?

In order for people to live to more of their biological potential, they must not die prematurely of diseases or afflictions which are, for the most part, preventable. In the United States, most of us will die before we reach our eightieth birthday. The Number One killer in America is heart disease. The Number Two killer is cancer. Other common afflictions which lead to untimely deaths include diabetes and the complications of osteoporosis.

With the knowledge we have today, there is much we can do to prevent, or at least delay for twenty or more years, the onset of these afflictions. Hard, empirical data from many scientific studies of population groups around the world support this statement. These population studies show that people from predominantly rural or agriculturally-based countries do not die prematurely from the same diseases as those from the industrialized countries. The causes of premature death in the United States, for instance, differ from what the people of rural China die of. In China, heart disease, cancer, and osteoporosis are minor afflictions which don't greatly influence the health of most of the people.

The people of rural China, however, do not have longer life expectancy rates than people in the United States. How do researchers explain this apparent contradiction? The explanation is simple. The Chinese people die prematurely of afflictions most of the industrialized countries have had under control for decades. The rural Chinese die of diseases associated with poverty, such as pneumonia, tuberculosis, and parasitic diseases. In a sense, it's ironic. Researchers are proposing that we achieve more of our biological life span potential of 120 years by following the lifestyles of the so-called non-industrialized people of the world. The only problem for such "non-industrialized people" is that the remarkable advances made in medical technology are, for the most part, not available to them.

So, the challenge is to combine the best parts of both worlds: (1) Adopt the diet and lifestyle of the less industrialized countries, and (2) take advantage of medical technology and education available in the more industrialized countries.

Now, let's talk about the things that cause too many Americans to die prematurely. The shame of the matter is that the diseases most commonly associated with the industrialized countries are all highly preventable. These diseases are, for the most part, brought on ourselves by what we put into our mouths. The irony of the situation is that, while we sit in front of our TV sets with bags of grease-glazed chips and boxes of *Little Debbie* bars, watching scenes of poor, malnourished people of Third World countries, we ourselves fail to admit or recognize that we, too, are a sadly malnourished society. The majority of people in modern industrialized countries like the United States consume more calories (too often empty calories) than needed daily. Many of the calories are nutrient poor. The human body, recognizing that the food consumed is lacking in nutrients, increases the appetite to obtain the missing nutrients. ***This cycle of eating more and more nutrient-poor foods in response to the body's demand for nutrients, leads to obesity and associated heart disease diabetes and cancer.***

VICIOUS CYCLE

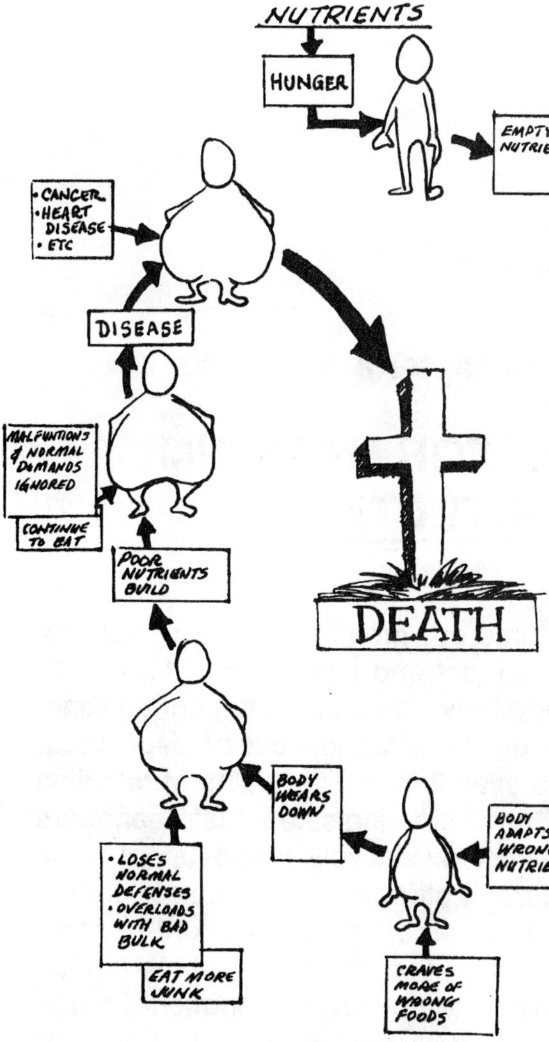

OF POOR NUTRIENT FOODS

Chapter 2

THE DIET FOR MAXIMUM PROTECTION

WHAT we put into our mouths can affect the way we sleep, think, act and feel. Certain foods can cause hyperactivity, others can fog our thinking, slow us down, make us feel dragged out or depressed. Behavior studies have even linked diet to acts of rebellion and delinquency. One study indicated that teenagers whose diets were almost exclusively made up of "junk foods" like hamburgers, hotdogs, potato chips, french fries, soda, candy, and other grease-packed, sugar-stuffed "garbage," were significantly more likely to participate in acts of rebellion, demonstrate delinquent behavior, and show decreased motivation to excel in school or work than those teenagers who ate healthier foods.

Diet has also been linked to depression, anxiety, and mental acuity. Certain foods can even affect how well we sleep at night. Most of us already know how foods with caffeine (such as coffee, tea, chocolate, or soda) affect us. Many people respond to such foods by becoming anxious, "wired", and unable to sleep. While some of us actually desire this effect (if we need to wake up, for instance), the long-term effect usually results in a dragged out feeling. Sugar can have a similar effect of shooting us up into a quick burst of energy, then dropping us down shortly afterward in an even lower "low." People who consume mostly heavy, high-fat foods are short-circuiting their energy supply and hampering much of their overall performance potential. Commercials which promote the fallacy that a chocolate candy bar will give an athlete more energy to perform should be removed. Be careful about how seriously you take TV commercials and other advertisements. Advertisers, aware that a larger percentage of the population today is interested in healthier foods, are now trying to promote their products in a way which makes them sound "healthy" or "natural," when, in reality, they are often false or distorted presentations. Even sugar has jumped in with ads suggesting that sugar is something "natural," and therefore (it is hopefully assumed), "good for you." Read labels when buying food products -- even in health food stores! Just because it says "healthy" or "nutrient rich" or "all natural" doesn't mean that it really is. Many cereals, for example, suggest in their packaging that they are good for you. But when you read the list of ingredients, they are loaded with fat and sugar. Sometimes the sugar comes in different disguises, such as "glucose," "fructose," "corn syrup," etc. Many of the so-called "healthy" cereals have actually had their natural nutrients crushed out of them during processing, then have had to have vitamins and minerals artificially added to make up for this loss. Such cereals are poor substitutes for the originally nutrient-rich grains we should be getting.

Poor dietary habits can dramatically increase your

risk of developing one or more of the four killer diseases (heart disease, cancer, osteoporosis, and diabetes), diet also plays a significant role in the prevention of such barriers to our longevity. A low-fat, low-protein, high-complex carbohydrate diet is the diet of choice for maximum protection against these destructive forces.

The Choice Foods

Include in this diet 5-7 servings per day of fruits and vegetables of all colors. Fruits and vegetables are low in fat and protein. They are also high in complex carbohydrates with its accompanying high-fiber content. Fruits and vegetables also have nutrient components which have been shown in research studies to have preventive action against heart disease and cancer.

Examples of desirable fruits to choose from are apples, bananas, oranges, pears, and cantaloupe. These are by no means the only desirable fruits. These fruits have a good blend of desirable fiber and antioxidant nutrients. Antioxidants help protect the body from damaging by-products of metabolism and respiration which contribute to heart disease and cancer.

Examples of desirable vegetables to choose from are carrots, broccoli, cauliflower, corn, green beans, and brussels sprouts. Many other vegetables are also beneficial. These vegetables are good sources of indoles, phthalides, fiber, and antioxidants. New research shows that these substances have a preventative effect on heart disease and cancer.

Eat at least two fruits and two vegetables daily. Consuming these quantities of fruits and vegetables will ensure an ample supply of the above-mentioned beneficial nutrients.

Protein: How Much Do You Need?

First, you must be aware that protein is an essential component of your body. Twenty to twenty-five percent of your body is composed of protein. But just how much do we actually need? In order to answer this question, you need to understand that the protein already in your body is re-usable. Protein is used in our bodies for growth and repair, and sometimes for energy production. When protein is broken down for these functions, its components, the amino acids (known as the "building blocks" of protein), can be reused at a later time when protein is required by the body again. The protein you consume is used over and over again. Some of the amino acids are used up in the growth and repair functions, but the rest are stored for later use.

Unless you are a growing child, a pregnant woman, or a burn victim, your protein needs are much more modest than you probably think. The RDA for protein is close to one gram for every three pounds of body weight per day. For most of us, this falls between 40 and 60 grams of protein per day. The average American diet includes more than 100 grams of protein per day. A small amount of protein can be stored in the liver as a reserve. All other protein consumed in excess of the storage capacity is broken down and stored as fat.

When you consume too much protein, excess nitrogen builds up and must be eliminated. Your body must be in nitrogen balance to function properly. Protein is processed in the liver. The waste products from protein breakdown in the liver are sent to the kidneys for elimination. The more protein you eat, the more work the liver and kidneys must do in order to eliminate the toxic by-products of protein breakdown.

As we consume more protein than our bodies require, the extra strain to process the toxic by-products takes its toll on many organs and systems of the body. The extra nitrogen circulating in the blood from excess protein breakdown causes the pH level to become more acidic. This acidic condition requires calcium and other minerals to be drawn from the bones and teeth to balance the pH of the blood. The wasting of calcium and other minerals to balance the blood promotes the development of osteoporosis.[1]

In addition to placing a tremendous workload on the liver and kidneys, excess protein has been shown in studies to increase the promotion of cancerous tumors and to suppress the function of the immune system in general. In 1939, Dr. Clive McCay of Cornell University demonstrated that rats fed low-protein diets lived almost 1-1/2 times longer than those fed a "normal" diet.[2] He later observed that the rats fed a protein-restricted diet had much less cancerous tumor development.[3]

Several studies conducted by members of Dr. T. Colin Campbell's research team at Cornell University have demonstrated that low-protein diets enhance the immune system by increasing the production of natural killer cells which destroy cancer cells.[4] Dr. Campbell has concluded that high-protein diets increase the enzymes which promote carcinogen production and bind these carcinogens to DNA, thus starting the growth of cancerous tumors. On the other hand, if you restrict your protein consumption, the cancer-promoting enzymes are greatly suppressed.[5]

The by-product of animal-based protein is uric acid. Excess uric acid in our system contributes to gout, kidney stones, and arthritis. Besides such damage done to our bodies, excess protein wears down and ages the body in general. If you want to look and feel older than your biological age, consume excess protein.

Vegetarianism

The understanding of the *Circulating Pool Theory* of amino acids has changed how the medical profession feels about the safety of vegetarian diets. It was mistakenly believed by doctors (not vegetarians) that humans had to consume complete proteins (proteins with all essential amino acids) at any one meal or else the proteins would be unusable. Research has so conclusively proven that this was never the case and that the circulating pool of amino acids in your body would provide any missing amino acids from a given food to make it a complete protein. Arthur Guyton, in his book, *The Physiology of the Body*, proved that humans are designed to function without ***any*** dietary protein for thirty days.[6]

We humans were originally designed for a diet of fruits and vegetables. The Bible describes a man named Daniel who practiced vegetarianism. He was taken into the king's palace and was offered a diet rich in meats and wine -- the diet shared and recommended by the king himself. But Daniel refused the meat and wine and requested vegetables only. But the king's servant worried over Daniel's decision, reasoning that such a diet would make him look pale and older than his years and that it would weaken him and make him sickly. But Daniel replied, "Please test your servants for ten days, and let them give us vegetables to eat and water to drink. Then let our countenances be examined before you, and the countenances of the young men who eat the portion of the king's delicacies; and as you see fit, so deal with your servants." (Daniel 1:12-13) And at the end of ten days, Daniel and those who had been served the vegetables and water only looked *better* than those who had eaten the king's meat. (Daniel 1:15) After only *ten days!*

We're simply not designed to eat meat. Our teeth are not canine teeth like those of a lion or tiger and our digestive tract in not equipped to digest proteins efficiently. Unlike the lion or tiger, our saliva contains enzymes to digest carbohydrates, not proteins. We also have too long of an intestinal tract to eat meat and other high-protein foods. Our digestive tract is close to 33 feet long, whereas a lion's digestive tract is only 7 to 10 feet long. Therefore, a lion can digest protein much more efficiently than a human being. Primates have similar digestive tracts to us, and they eat bamboo shoots and bananas. They do not eat meat. Meat and digestive by-products of meat also put off carcinogens like nitrates and nitrosomes. Bacon, for instance, is very high in nitrates and is considered one of the more cancer-causing foods.

Though this may surprise some of you, chicken is actually meat. Chicken is sometimes worse to eat than beef, especially after what is done to them during captivity these days. If you want to eat poultry, it's better to eat turkey than chicken, as they are usually free range running birds.

Food Combinations for Maximum Nutrient Absorption

How we combine different foods makes a difference in how well our body absorbs and activates the nutrients of each. Combine vegetables and starch foods together to get the most benefit in a proper nutrient balance. Beans and rice have been used for decades in healthy meal selections. Beans and rice provide ample protein for growth and maintenance needs, while being low in fat and high in complex carbohydrates. Vegetable soup with rice, noodles, beans, or potatoes is another fine choice. Numerous other combinations are possible without using high-fat, high-protein food items.

Food Preparation

How we prepare our foods is very important if we want the greatest nutritional benefit. Don't overcook fruits and vegetables, as this boils the nutrients out of them. Soups or stews are an exception since most nutrients boiled out can be rescued in the broth (especially if cooked with a cover to seal in nutrients trying to escape through steam).

Frying foods in oils also depreciates their nutritional value. During the cooking process, the oils absorb into the foods and increase the fat content. Re-heating fried foods is even worse. It *doubles* their negative effect.

The process of evaporation during cooking can also deplete foods of their nutrients.

The rule of thumb for fruits and vegetables is to eat them as close to their natural state as possible.

The Importance of Water

Most people neglect to drink sufficient amounts of water. No matter how many other fluids you drink, there is nothing that can quite take the place of water in your system. Water plays a tremendous part in every chemical reaction that takes place in our bodies. The reactions which take place while we eat, sleep, and move all involve the use of water. Without water in our system, we would die in a matter of days. The only other more essential element for us is air.

The amount of water we drink not only affects the efficient functioning or our internal organs, but also influences the texture of our skin. Water purges and purifies. It washes out impurities in our blood, resulting in an improved complexion which is clearer, smoother and more moisture-balanced.

Water is the "oil" we need to keep everything in our system lubricated and running efficiently.

Low-Protein Food Choices

A good, low-protein diet should include one ounce of raw, unsalted nuts or seeds (pumpkin seeds and almonds are excellent choices) 3-4 times per week. Do not eat the nuts and seeds in addition to beef or chicken, but as a replacement for these food items. If you eat nuts, seeds and meat, you will be getting excess protein in your diet. Contrary to popular belief, chicken and fish are meat. Count the protein grams in your diet daily for two weeks. Compare your gram count with the desirable range. Most likely, you will have to adjust your protein grams downward.

Low-Fat Food Choices

High-fat diets promote heart disease and cancer. Eliminate the high-fat items in your diet. Read labels. Count the fat grams in all the foods you eat. Reduce the use of dairy products, as they contribute to many of your health problems.

Milk, cheese and eggs are high in fat and protein. You do not need dairy products to prevent osteoporosis. High-protein diets are the main cause of osteoporosis. There can be a small place for dairy products in your diet. Use low- or no-fat dairy products only.

The worst high-fat foods are butter, oils, gravies, snack foods, crackers, and desserts. These foods are usually loaded with both obvious and hidden fats.

Saltines, *Ritz* crackers, and most other crackers are loaded with hidden saturated fats. Eliminate these and other snack foods from your diet.

Cookies and desserts are typically loaded with saturated fats. Salad dressings and oils are mostly fat. A tablespoon of oil can contain up to 14 grams of fat. Choose no-fat or low-fat salad dressing. Many new choices have come on the market recently. It is much easier today to choose low- or no-fat alternatives for your desert choices.

Remember to read the labels on food packages. Count the fat grams in your daily diet for two weeks. If you do this, you will know the fat gram content of the foods you regularly eat. Keep the fat content of your diet to no more than 15 percent. An easier guide is to eat no more than 20-30 grams of fat per day.

High-Complex Carbohydrates

Complex carbohydrates are the "food of choice." The fiber contained in the complex carbohydrates causes a slow release of glucose into the intestines. This slow release of glucose from carbohydrate digestion helps your insulin to function more efficiently in controlling your blood glucose levels. When your glucose levels are under control, you feel more satisfied and free of hunger pains. As mentioned earlier, fruits and vegetables are good sources of the complex carbohydrates. Whole grain pastas are also excellent sources of the complex carbohydrates. Include baked potatoes, brown rice, and whole grain pastas into your daily diet. Be careful about which toppings you put on them. There are many low-fat butter and topping substitutes to choose from.

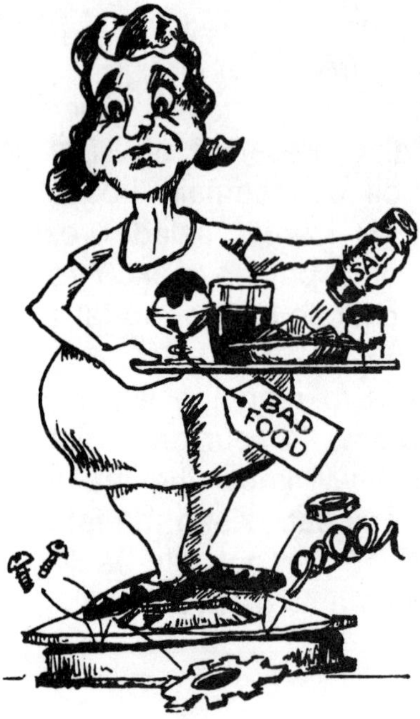

Re-Evaluating Food

Many people have lost track of *why* we eat. Food is meant to give us strength, energy, and fuel to operate. Our body demands certain nutrients and lubricants, and, as was demonstrated in the "Vicious Cycle" illustration in Chapter One, will continue to crave the missing ingredients until sufficiently satisfied. If we continue to pour in all the wrong things, our body will continue to have cravings in its attempt to fulfill its basic needs. Until you begin to consume more appropriate foods, you will have diet problems.

Food is also meant to be *enjoyed*. Don't think you have to go through the rest of your life eating foods which are unpleasant to you. Healthy foods can actually become more enjoyable than junk food, once you've adapted to them. We can actually re-train our tastebuds, you know. If, for instance, you have been a "junk food junkie" most of your life, you might find "healthy" foods undesirable at first. Therefore, once you make the decision to take better care of yourself and increase your life span, you may have to go through a "cold turkey" period of adjustment. For some people, this period is very brief. For others, it may take a little longer. One thing which might make this period more successful is to think of all the horrible things your junk food diet is doing to your system, and then convince yourself that these bad foods are really quite unappealing -- even abhorrent. Much of your success will have to come from what you put into your *mind.*

Table 2.1 highlights some desirable foods. Foods in the table have been selected for their high nutrient content in more than one category. Eat foods listed in this table daily.

TABLE 2.1
HEALTHFUL FOOD CHOICES

DESCRIPTION	PROTEIN (gm)	FAT (gm)	CARBO'S (gm)	FIBER (gm)
Apples, Raw 1 ea.	.4	.8	32	6.5
Bananas, Raw 1 ea.	1.2	.5	26.7	3.26
Orange, Raw 1 ea.	1.2	.2	15.4	2.97
Figs, Dried 10 ea.	5.7	2.2	122	24
Cantaloupe 1/2 ea.	2.4	.7	22.3	2.67
Pears 1 ea.	.7	.7	25.1	4.98
Green Beans 1 cup	2.4	.4	9.9	3.13
Broccoli 1 cup	2.6	.3	4.6	3.34
Brussels Sprouts 1 cup	6	.8	13.5	5.62
Cabbage 1 cup	1	.1	3.8	1.62
Carrots 1 ea.	.7	.1	7.3	2.03
Corn 1 cup	5	.1	33.6	7.7
Cauliflower 1 cup	2.4	.1	5.8	3.3
Eggplant 1 cup	1.3	.4	10.6	6
Peas 1 cup	8.2	.4	22.8	15.2
Tofu 1/2 cup	18.8	5	2.9	2.2
Spinach Raw 1 cup	1.6	.2	2	2.3
Potato Baked/Skin 1 ea.	4.7	.2	51	4.4
Sweet Potato 1 ea.	2	.1	27.2	2.96
Grt Northern Beans 1 cup	14	1.1	38.2	12.4
Kidney Beans 1 cup	14.5	.9	41.8	20
Brown Rice 1 cup	4.9	1.2	49.7	3.9

Chapter 3

EXERCISE

What Part Does It Play In the Equation?

ALL the preventative strategies I recommended in the previous chapters are only half as effective without the inclusion of exercise into the equation. Exercise must play a predominant role in your total health plan. Exercise energizes and enhances many of the bodily functions.

The human body is designed for movement. The utilization of blood sugar, the strengthening of bones and muscles, and the effectiveness of the immune system are all enhanced by regular, sustained physical activity. High or low blood sugar, weak or atrophied bones and muscles, and an ineffective immune system can result from physical inactivity. You can follow a low-fat, low-protein diet and achieve good health, but you will never reach super health without the inclusion of a regular, sustained exercise program.

Exercise has many far-reaching consequences on physical and mental systems of the body. Exercise can aid in the control of diabetes, strengthen bones and muscles, and play a part in the prevention of heart disease and cancer. It can aid the digestive system by increasing bowel activity and can act as a stress reliever, thus calming the central nervous system.

In this chapter, I will describe some of the benefits a regular exercise program can contribute to your maximum health potential. I will explain the benefits of aerobic exercise programs as well as the benefits of other exercise programs. The benefits of one of these exercise programs is not commonly appreciated. I think I will catch many of you by surprise with this one. Flexibility is another important exercise factor often overlooked. Finally, I will outline the hydration and fuel requirements essential to achieve maximum performance for the weekend athlete, as well as the competitive athlete.

Not all exercises are alike. Different exercises work differently on different parts of the body and for different purposes. I will try to present a basic outline of some of the more common types of exercise.

Aerobics

Long before Jane Fonda or even Dr. Kenneth Cooper, the so-called "father of aerobics," started to preach the benefits of aerobic exercise, Jack LaLanne and his dog, Happy, showed us the benefits of regular aerobic exercise on his daily television show in the sixties. I talked about this man in Chapter 1. He was obviously extremely fit as a result of his regular aerobic exercise program. Today, Jack is in his early 80s and can probably still outperform most of us in any aerobic exercise pro-

REGULAR EXERCISE

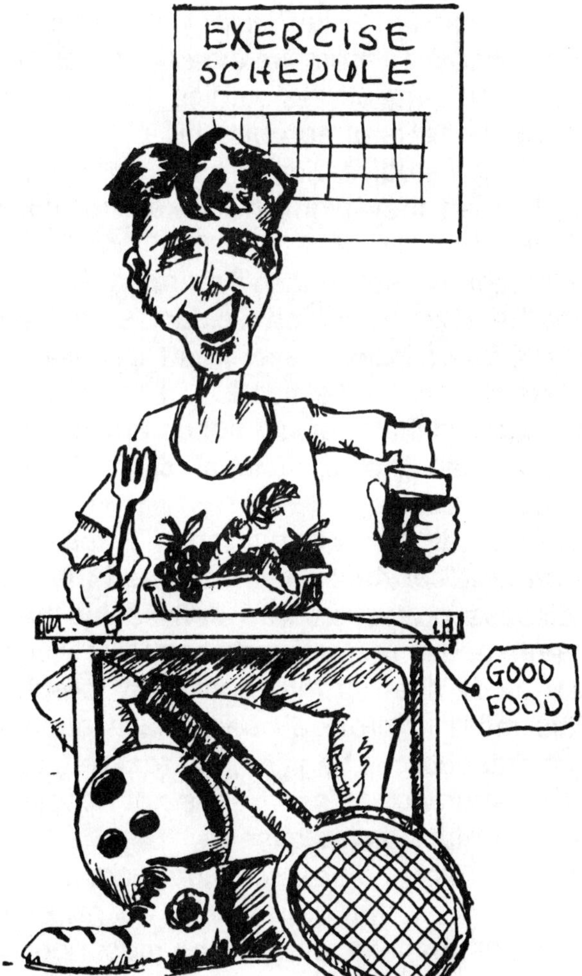

DOES THE TRICK

gram. We could all enjoy the health benefits Jack has derived if we would take the time and effort needed to reach his level of fitness.

The good news is that exercise intensity does not have to be extreme to achieve heart health. Walking, hiking, or even casual biking give you protection from heart disease almost as much as strenuous aerobic workouts. Many of the early fitness studies that were cited as evidence of the benefits of aerobics did not focus on aerobics at all. These studies didn't include running, cycling, or rowing. Instead they highlighted walking, hiking and even ticket taking.

That's right. A 1953 British Transport Worker Study showed that the ticket takers on England's double decker buses showed lower incidence of heart disease than the sedentary bus drivers. Investigation of the habits of the ticket takers showed that they did not do any extra aerobic exercise other than the occasional stair climbing and walking on the buses.

Another study in 1966, published in the *Journal of the American Medical Association*, showed that substantial heart disease protection was derived by the participants who engaged in recreational sports like walking and hiking. The study showed that additional aerobic exercise did little more to provide heart health protection. I think the general public is beginning to realize that the "no pain, no gain" approach to exercise is not necessary and can even be harmful in some cases.

Take time to plan an exercise program that fits your lifestyle. Any program you do regularly will give you most of the heart health benefits of even the most rigorous aerobic program. A study done by Arthur Leon, M.D., of the University of Minnesota, showed that men who burned on average only 285 calories per day during activities such as walking, gardening, or fishing, derived as much heart benefit as those who burned twice as many calories doing strenuous aerobic exercises. Do anything. Just do *something.*

Most of the heart health benefits of exercise are derived from small to moderate amounts. But if you are determined to squeeze out that extra 10-15% heart health benefit from exercise, then you have to follow certain rules. A study involving participants exercising at 65, 75 and 85 percent of maximum heart rates showed different heart health results. Those participants who exercised at heart maximum rates of 75 percent or more, showed elevation in their beneficial HDL levels. Those at the 65 percent maximum heart rate did not show elevated HDL levels.

The study also showed that those who only reached the 75 percent heart rate level were still able to lower their harmful LDL levels.[1] Obviously, more studies are needed in this area to come to a final conclusion regarding the different health benefits of the various exercise intensity levels. Meanwhile, enough evidence is present to recognize the benefits of exercising at at least 75 percent of your maximum heart rate.

Resistance/Strengthening Exercises

Resistance-type exercises (exercises which strengthen muscles and bones, such as weight-lifting exercises) are one of the most important, though often misunderstood, types of exercise necessary for longevity. If you follow all the dietary and lifestyle changes I recommend in this book, you will go far to extend your usable life span. But what about the frame which has to support this longer-lived person?

If you live past seventy years, your skeletal and muscular system must be in better than average condition in order to prevent minor accidents from crippling or end-ing your life. It is important that you regularly participate in resistance exercises to ensure that your musculoskeletal system is strong enough to withstand the bumps and scrapes of life.

The time to strengthen your foundation is now. If you are young, it's the perfect time to begin strengthening the structure. If you are elderly, it's not too late to begin. Numerous studies conducted on the elderly show that weight resistance training is just as effective on the elderly at building muscle mass as it is on the young. In other words, a person in his or her seventies can build muscle size and strength just about as well as a teenager can.

How do resistance exercises help your muscles and bones? The act of lifting a weight involves not only muscles, but bones as well. When a muscle is flexed, as in lifting an object, the bones attached to it are put under stress. When bones and muscles are put under stress they react to stress by growing denser and stronger. They respond this way in order to adapt to stress. Repeated stress in this way will cause the bones and muscles to continue to adapt by growing denser and stronger.

Your need for a strong musculoskeletal system is manifold. As we get older, the spaces between our vertebrae begin to narrow due to gravity. Strong back and abdominal muscles can help prevent much of this spinal compression by shielding the back from the effects of gravity. Strong abdominal and lower back muscles can also help prevent many back injuries. Strengthening the muscles surrounding your joints, such as those in the shoulder and knee, can go a long way in preventing many of the frequent injuries which plague these two joints.

My friend, Bob, who is a well-conditioned athlete, has been plagued with numerous shoulder and knee injuries. The most severe injury was to his shoulder, requiring surgery and years of therapy to get moderate use of it back. While he was recuperating from shoulder surgery, he decided to compete in running competitions. About the time he began to enjoy the training and races, he injured his knee. It seemed as if he couldn't win.

Through rehabilitation on his shoulder, Bob realized what his problem was. He said that if he had only strengthened the muscles around his shoulder and knee before demanding so much from them, he could probably have avoided his injuries in the first place. The point is, you don't have to be a competitive athlete to injure a muscle or joint. You can injure yourself during even the simplest exercises, such as walking or an aerobics class. Before starting an exercise program for the health of it, it's a good idea to determine which muscles and joints will be most affected, then strengthen them beforehand in order to prevent injury. If you are already involved in an exercise program, add weight training to enhance your performance and also to add an extra measure of protection from injury.

Flexibility

Most of us have been told repeatedly about the virtues of stretching to prevent injury. Proper stretching has been found to reduce the incidence of injury. However, in our quest to become more and more flexible, some stretching enthusiasts appear to have taken it too far. Recent studies are showing a backlash of injuries associated with stretching muscles and ligaments too far.

First of all, stretching should be done *after* your body is warmed up, not when you are cold. More injuries occur because we try to stretch when the muscles are cold and inflexible than if we didn't stretch at all. In the typical scenario, we are in a hurry to start exercising, so we decide to force our chins to our knees or our palms to the floor. Pain is no obstacle. We just know that if we can reach these marks we will have performed our duty. This is exactly the time we are likely to cause an injury, rather than prevent it.

It's important to warm up for at least fifteen to twenty minutes before stretching. Some people confuse warm-up exercises with stretching exercises. They're *not* the same thing. Warm-ups might include walking around a bit, doing calisthenics (not the same as *stretching* exercises), isometrics, a brief jog around the room, or even just moving about until your body feels "warmed." You should raise your body temperature a degree or two in order to increase the circulation to the muscles you are trying to stretch. Increased blood flow to the muscles will help them become less rigid and more flexible. The important thing to remember during your warm-up (as well as during your stretching), is to *go slowly*. **Never** try to rush your muscles into a warm-up! Not only will a hurried warm-up risk injury, but you will also lose much of the benefit to your muscles. This doesn't mean you have to take two hours out of your busy day to warm up. It just means you need to learn to be kinder to your muscles and bones. Be sensitive to their movement and how each muscle and bone responds to that movement. Learn to get in touch with what your body is telling you. If it screams when you do a particular exercise, listen. Don't ignore the scream. There's a difference between a "scream" in your body and a "whimper of protest." A whimper of protest may mean that your body is simply unaccustomed to a new or increased movement which it really should make. But a scream can be a warning of approaching damage. Think of it this way. If your child moans and complains when you ask him to do something he's not used to doing, you'll still make him do it if you know it's good for him to do. You also happen to know that he'll get used to the new activity soon enough and will probably even learn to enjoy it. But if your child screams with complete terror (not stubbornness) and trembling, you had better at least listen and find out what the problem is. Just as you need to truly listen to your children, you need to truly listen to your body.

How far you try to stretch is also important. The main purpose of stretching is to elongate and increase the flexibility of a muscle or group of muscles. If a muscle is more flexible, it is less likely that a sudden movement or extension will cause an injury. It is important, however, not to *overstretch*. Recent studies have shown that athletes who continue to push their muscles into increased flexibility have a *greater* incidence of injury.[2] Increasing the range of motion of certain muscles and tendons can increase the chances of injuring certain joints, such as the knee. When you overstretch the quadricep muscles on the front of your leg, you also stretch the tendons which support the knee. The knee is not a very stable joint to begin with. When the muscles and tendons supporting it are overstretched, the knee joint begins to get "sloppy." The more out-of-range movement the knee is allowed to have, the greater the chances of injury.

When we were children, we were naturally flexible. As we grow older, our muscles and joints get stiffer and less flexible. Our goal in stretching is to come closer to the flexibility we knew as children. We don't want to overflex, as this may cause us to lose needed support for our joints. It is especially dangerous to do lots of stretching exercises without any muscle-strengthening exercises. If you fail to first strengthen your musculoskeletal structure, your joints become sloppy and more prone to injury. Your joints need *support* to keep in place and work properly. It's the job of your muscles and ligaments to give this support.

Flexibility is good, but don't overdo it.

After you warm up, you can then begin your stretching routine with less fear of injuring yourself. Don't forget to stretch afterward as well. Stretching after a workout will prevent muscle soreness. It also helps to eliminate lactic acid buildup (evidenced by a burning sensation in your muscles) and, since you are more flexible after exercise than before, you will be able to stretch further with greater ease and therefore increase your overall flexibility.

Stress-Reduction Exercises

The American Heritage Dictionary defines stress as "a mentally or emotionally disruptive or disquieting influence; [or] an applied force or system of forces that tends to strain or deform a body."

Some degree of stress is an inescapable influence for most of us. In the fast-paced society we live in today, it is especially difficult to avoid. Nonetheless, we needn't let stress get the best of us -- though it will certainly try to do just that. Stress puts a heavy strain on muscles, bones, ligaments, the skin, the heart, the internal organs, and, in fact, every part of our body. If stress is not kept under control, it will eventually begin to tear us down -- physically, emotionally, and mentally. As was mentioned in Chapter 1, we are made up of body, soul and spirit. Therefore, if our soul (mind, emotions, will) is in distress (under stress), it naturally affects our body. The same is true when we place our body under too much stress, as when we run ourselves to the ground with overwork, overplay, or lack of rest. If our body is overtired (stressed), it affects how we respond emotionally, mentally and spiritually (ie, we start getting short-tempered, irritable, apathetic, wired, or unable to think clearly). Along these same lines, it is clear that physical exercise actually helps us deal with and reduce emotional or mental stress.

Stress comes in many different packages. There's physical stress, emotional stress, and mental stress. Most of us usually think of emotional stress when we hear the word, probably because this is one of the hardest forms of stress to deal with. But think about the mental stress you experience when you work on a business project for hours. You come home physically exhausted, even though you've been at your desk all day. You're physically exhausted because your body has reacted to the mental and emotional stress of the day. In addition, your body has actually been under a strain just from having to stay in one bent position over a desk for so long without relief. This is why it's important to take time out during your work day to walk around and do a few warm-up exercises.

Any physical exercise will help reduce stress. This includes aerobic workouts, calisthenics, isometrics, warm-ups, stretching, and weight-lifting/resistance exercises. But there are certain exercises which are particularly helpful in teaching us how to relax. Some of these exercises include muscle-tightening movements alternated with muscle-releasing reactions (tensing muscles, then relaxing). This kind of exercise makes us more aware of what's happening in our body and gives us greater control over its reactions. Another stress-reduction exercise involves deep breathing awareness combined with very slow movements of the body, as with raising your arm up and down while in a comfortable supine position, noting how each muscle fiber feels during movement. You might also want to try listening to some very soothing instrumental music while lying in a quiet place and concentrating on making every part of your body relax.

You will discover that, the more fit you are physically, the better able you are to handle stress.

Rehabilitative Exercises

If you have experienced an injury of some sort, you may be able to speed up your healing process, or even improve your physical condition beyond what it was before the injury, by doing rehabilitative exercises. These kinds of exercises, however, must be closely monitored by your physician and should be under the instruction of a physical or recreational therapist. Such professionals are able to diagnose your current capabilities for movement. Trying to exercise too soon after an injury, or doing the wrong kinds of exercises, can cause serious damage. However, since not all doctors fully understand every aspect of bone, muscle and ligament rehabilitation, you may want to get two or three different medical opinions before resigning to a sedentary lifestyle.

Our bones are active, living tissue. If we can improve the structure of our muscles and ligaments through exercise, what's to stop us from improving our bones? Also, keep in mind that our bones need the support of our muscles and ligaments to function most effectively. So, the weaker and more unstable our muscles and ligaments are, the less support we will have for our bones. If your bones are out of alignment, for instance, you cannot expect them to regain total stability if your muscles are too weak to hold them in place.

There are countless testimonies of people who have dramatically improved, and, in many cases, entirely overcome, their medical handicap through exercise. Even people with muscular dystrophy have been known to improve their functioning ability with exercise -- particularly with pool/water therapy.

Diet For Maximum Performance

If you are eating the wrong proportions of carbohydrates, proteins and fats, or eating them at the wrong times, you could be hindering your exercise performance. With the dizzying amount of diet programs available today, most of us are confused as to which program is best for us. Allow me to unravel some of the mystery centered around diet and exercise performance.

Whether you're a weekend warrior or a professional athlete, diet can help make or break your performance goals. There are biochemical rules and pathways that the human body follows. The pathways concerning the contraction of muscles and the storage of the fuel they need is of prime concern to those who want to achieve maximum performance.

Understanding the Biochemical Rules

A biology professor of mine once said that "we are nothing more than a bag of chemical reactions." This idea is highlighted in the anatomy of a muscle contraction. Our main quick energy source for movement or muscle contraction comes from a compound called ATP. This compound is found within the muscle cells. When we require movement, ATP is broken down by enzymes releasing the energy needed to cause muscles to contract.

In the early stages of exercise, your stores of ATP are depleted quickly. The cells then call on glycogen stores to reproduce more ATP. Glycogen is the storage form of the glucose we receive from the foods we eat. As this process continues, the glycogen is used up, producing a by-product called *lactic acid*. As the lactic acid builds up in the cells, it begins to retard muscle contraction. It is this buildup of lactic acid that causes the burning sensation in your muscles.

This process takes place within the cell without the use of oxygen. It is called the *anaerobic pathway* of energy production. This form of energy is your quick-start energy, good for only two or three minutes of activity before lactic acid cripples muscle contraction. The anaerobic pathway is necessary for quick starts of muscle contraction before the heart and lungs can be brought into play.

If you continue exercising beyond two or three minutes, oxygen enters the scene to combine with the lactic acid to produce glycogen, which your body can convert into ATP. This process is called the *aerobic pathway.* Now you understand the meaning of the term "aerobics." Aerobic (requiring "air") exercises involve a slow-to-medium pace workout where the heart and lungs are able to provide enough oxygen to the working muscles.

Aerobic exercises do not *cause* an overload of lactic acid. While engaging in aerobic exercises, the lactic acid produced is able to combine with oxygen from the lungs to produce glycogen. With the aerobic pathway of energy, we can exercise almost indefinitely if enough oxygen is available to the muscle cells.

All these chemical reactions require an outside fuel source. The carbohydrates, proteins and fats from your diet, along with water and oxygen, combine to provide the fuel needed. The premier fuel is carbohydrates. Carbohydrates are broken down in the digestive system into glucose, then stored in the liver and muscles in the form of glycogen.

Now that we know carbohydrates are the body's primary fuel, it is equally important to know what kind of carbohydrates the body prefers. There are basically two types of carbohydrates: simple and complex. The simple carbohydrates, such as those found in candies, cookies, and refined flour products, are devoid of fiber or nutrients of any significant value. These carbohydrates do not have the necessary raw materials to sustain vigorous exercise for any length of time. Most people realize that the simple carbohydrates found in candies and refined flour products don't have beneficial nutrients, but most of us don't realize that these simple carbohydrates actually use up existing supplies of vitamins and minerals in order to be digested and assimilated. All foods eaten require the use of existing nutrients in order to be digested and assimilated. When you eat nutrient-rich foods, your body absorbs more vitamins and minerals during the digestion process than what you use up. When the carbohydrates in your diet are mainly simple carbohydrates, you are actually draining you system of needed nutrients.

A diet consisting mainly of simple carbohydrates will result in early fatigue and poor performance. This is one of the main reasons for unexplained exercise plateaus and poor performance. Simple carbohydrates are absorbed into the bloodstream rapidly, causing spikes and then dips in your blood sugar levels. These spikes and dips sap your energy reserves in an effort to stabilize your blood sugar levels. Your brain needs an even level of blood sugar in order to function properly. When the blood sugar levels from simple carbohydrates spike and dip, a condition called hypoglycemia (which means low blood sugar) exists, causing lack of concentration and fatigue.

In contrast, complex carbohydrates provide a steady, even flow of glucose into the bloodstream. Complex carbohydrates, by nature, have larger quantities of fiber than simple carbohydrates. When fiber-rich foods enter the small intestines, where most nutrient absorption takes place, the fiber slows down the release of glucose into the bloodstream. This slow release stabilizes the blood glucose levels. Stable blood glucose levels are the most efficient way to provide fuel to the working muscles. Complex carbohydrates also contain much greater quantities of vitamins and minerals than are used up in the process of digestion and assimilation. These nutrients gained from the consumption of complex carbohydrates are used as catalysts in the chemical reactions that take place in the body to produce the energy needed for exercise.

Another factor that comes into play in the use of carbohydrates for fuel is called the glycemic effect of the food. The speed at which a carbohydrate is broken down into glucose for absorption into the bloodstream is of major importance in how you feel and how you perform. Carbohydrates which are broken down rapidly into glucose will raise your blood glucose rapidly. This rapid rise will lead to a corresponding rapid fall in glucose levels, usually one to two hours later.

Many exercise authorities recommend eating your pre-exercise meal two or more hours before your workout or match. If that meal consists of carbohydrates which raise glucose levels rapidly, with their corresponding rapid fall, you will begin your workout feeling tired and sluggish. If your glucose metabolism is not in optimal condition then you may also experience lightheadedness and cold sweats. As you can see, this is not the way to start an exercise workout. At best, you will be working with a severe handicap to your performance.

Your pre-exercise meal should consist of carbohydrates which are converted into glucose in the blood at a slow, steady pace. If you eat these types of carbohydrates, your blood glucose levels will remain constant well into your workout. Researchers have created an index to rate how rapidly foods are converted to glucose in the blood. This rating system is called the Glycemic Index. Simply put, the higher the rating a food has, the faster it is converted into glucose in the blood.

Researchers have discovered that the speed of conversion of a carbohydrate to glucose does not follow simple guidelines. You might assume that all simple carbohydrates cause a rapid rise in glucose levels and all complex carbohydrates cause a slow, steady rise. They discovered that actual glucose (directly ingested) causes the fastest rise in glucose levels when consumed, but that white bread and carrots were converted into blood glucose almost as rapidly. They also discovered that most fruits, which are simple carbohydrates, are converted slowly into blood glucose. One exception to that rule is bananas, which are converted rapidly. On the other hand, beans, lentils, yogurt, and most fruits are on the slow converting end of the Glycemic Index.

Many factors appear to play a part in the conversion speed of foods to blood glucose. For example, the digestibility of the carbohydrates in a food and their interactions with proteins greatly affect the rate at which they are converted into glucose in the blood. In addition, the amounts and kinds of fat, sugar and fiber in the food influence the speed of conversion.[3]

Table 3.1 highlights the general range of the glycemic affect of some selected foods. Foods in the high range on the table are converted rapidly into blood glucose. Foods at the bottom of the table are converted at a much slower rate.

TABLE 3.1
GLYCEMIC INDEX

FOOD ITEM	RATE OF GLUCOSE CONVERSION
Glucose	Very High
White Bread	(Worst)
Corn Flakes	
Carrots	High
Russet Potatoes	
Rice	
Bananas	
Whole Grain Bread	Medium
New Potatoes	
All-Bran Cereal	
Kidney beans	
Shredded Wheat Cereal	
Spaghetti	
Raisins	
Orange Juice	Low
Ice Cream	
Corn	
Sucrose (Table Sugar)	
Potato Chips	
Oatmeal	
Sweet Potatoes	
Navy Beans	
Peas	
Grapes, Oranges	
Garbanzo & Lima Beans	Very Low
Milk	(Best)
Apples, Pears, Cherries	
Peaches, Plums, Grapefruit	
Lentils	
Fructose (Fruit Sugar)	
Soybeans, Peanuts	

Source: The relationship between food and blood sugar, Nutrition and the MD, July 1984

Your diet should consist of 60 to 70 percent carbohydrates for maximum health and performance. These carbohydrates should be mostly of the complex variety. The simple carbohydrates in your diet should consist mainly of fruits. (Sugar is a simple carbohydrate; this is not a good choice. Most fruits, however, are also simple carbohydrates, and fruits *are* a good choice.) Your pre-exercise meal should contain at least 50 percent of its carbohydrates from the slow glucose release portion of *Table 3.1* to maintain a steady blood glucose level during exercise.

You are now aware of the benefits of eating complex carbohydrates with a low glycemic index during your pre-exercise meal. These carbohydrates will charge up your liver and muscle cells with the needed fuel for maximum performance. If proper time is not available before exercise, or the foods you need are not available for a pre-exercise meal, another good source of the necessary complex carbohydrates are *glucose polymers.* In essence, these glucose polymers are complex carbohydrates derived from a form of corn starch easily assimilated and digested. If you look at *Table 3.1*, you will see that corn is on the low end of the Glycemic Index.

Several new products on the market contain glucose polymers. Twin Labs is one of the companies which produces such products. Two of the products they produce are called, *Carboplex* and *Carbo Fuel.* Twin Labs takes their sports formulation one step further to enhance the speed and efficiency of their complex carbohydrates: they add fructose to their formulation.

Table 3.1 indicates that fructose is at the very bottom of the Glycemic Index. Earlier, I mentioned that the foods we eat are converted into glucose and then stored in the form of glycogen. This glycogen is stored in two primary sites: the liver and the muscles. Fructose, or fruit sugar, has the ability to restore the glycogen in your liver faster than any other type of food. If you use *Carbo Fuel* before and during exercise, you will recharge your liver glycogen stores at a rapid pace, thus fueling your continued exercise.

Glycogen = fuel for energy

Many advances have been made in today's sports supplements. The trick is for you to choose the most beneficial one to meet your goals. Many popular sports drinks such as *Gatorade* and *Exceed* have several properties which make them less than ideal choices to enhance your sports performance. Most of the popular sports drinks contain too much sodium and too many simple sugars.

After exercise, carbohydrates are just as essential. When you have finished your exercise routine, it is time to start thinking about replenishing the energy stores depleted. Timing is everything. Fifteen minutes to an hour after exercise is ideal for replenishing the carbohydrates used up in exercise. Just about everything you eat during this period will be used to replenish depleted glycogen stores. If you eat carbohydrates during this time period, your liver and muscle glycogen will be filled to maximum capacity. If you wait longer than this time period to replenish used glycogen stores, your liver and muscles will not be as receptive to storing as much glycogen. A study performed in 1988 by Ivy and colleagues found that when carbohydrate consumption was delayed for two hours or longer after exercise, muscle glycogen stores were filled only one-third as much as when carbohydrates were ingested immediately after training.[4] What this means to you is that the same amount of calories eaten at different times will be stored differently. Carbohydrates consumed after the highly receptive time period of two hours following exercise may not all be used to replace used glycogen in the liver and muscles. The carbohydrates and fats consumed after the liver and muscle cells stop refilling supplies are then stored as fat. This is an important fact to remember if you are trying to lose excess fat. Eat your big carbohydrate meal as soon as possible after your exercise routine and very little of the calories will be stored as fat.

Now you must eat the right foods at the right time, or you will hinder your exercise ability. If liver and muscle glycogen stores are not filled to capacity, you cannot expect to have the endurance to last for any prolonged exercise event.

Complex carbohydrates = steady energy flow

Simple carbohydrates = short-lived energy flow

Exercising with less than optimal glycogen stores can have very negative consequences. The body needs fuel to perform any kind of work. The ideal fuel source is glycogen from fully-loaded muscles and the liver. If these sources are not available, the body will break down fat and protein stores to get its needed fuel.

Fat is an inefficient source of fuel for the muscles. Only about 5 percent of stored fat can be converted into glucose. The glycerol portion of triglycerides can be used to synthesize glucose in a process called *gluconeogenesis.* On the other hand, this same process can convert about 50 percent of your stored protein to produce glucose for fuel.[5] You can see that protein is a much more efficient source of energy than fat. Unfortunately, the preferred source of protein is your muscle tissue.

To summarize carbohydrates' role, it is the primary

fuel for activity. Low Glycemic Index carbohydrates should be used to fill the glycogen stores of the liver and muscles. Consume carbohydrates as quickly as possible after strenuous exercise in order to refill the storage banks as completely as possible. Spare the protein in your muscles by exercising with a full load of carbohydrates.

Fat as an Energy Source

If carbohydrates are the primary fuel for exercise, then fat should be considered a significant secondary fuel source. Muscles and the liver have only limited ability to store glycogen for fuel. About 1-1/2 to 2 hours after you start strenuous exercise your glycogen supplies are used up. When the glycogen stores are gone, the body switches to burning fat. The fatty acid components of the fat are broken down and burned as fuel to power the muscles. Actually, some of your glycogen stores are kept in reserve for nervous system and brain function. If all your glycogen were used up in exercise activity, you would be rendered unconscious.

A long-distance run or a prolonged tennis match will rely heavily on your fat stores for fuel in the later stages of the event. Unconditioned athletes can feel the switch from burning carbohydrates to burning fat as a fuel. The term "hitting the wall" has been used to describe the feeling you get when you run out of glycogen fuel during an athletic event. This description is used because you literally feel as if you are trying to move your body through a wall with every effort you make.

Unfortunately, switching from muscle and liver stores of glycogen to burning fat for fuel is clumsy and inefficient. When such a switch occurs, your energy level and attention span may dip until your body makes the adjustment.

Here's a tip to increase your exercise ability and

performance: the more often you switch from burning glycogen to burning fat, the more efficient the transition becomes. If you train several times a week with durations of more than an hour, you will regularly be using fat as an energy source during your workout. You don't have to be a long-distance runner to achieve the benefits of burning fat as a fuel. A two-hour tennis match achieves the same goal.

What actually happens when you exercise in excess of an hour is that you burn fat as well as burning carbohydrates. This is called the carbohydrate-sparing effect of fat. When you are efficient at burning fat as a fuel, more of your carbohydrates are spared for later use in the event, thus giving you an extended source of energy.

The Benefits of Extended Duration Exercise

There are significant health benefits to exercising in excess of one hour on a regular basis. Have you noticed how long distance runners usually appear? Most of them are very thin. If you are not aware of this, go to a long-distance event in your area and take a look at the contestants. It will be obvious that they are very efficient at burning fat as a fuel.

If you exercise regularly long enough to use fat as a fuel, you will lose significant amounts of body fat. If one of your main goals in exercising is to lose weight, then you should exercise for longer periods of time rather than more frequent 20-minute sessions. For example, walking briskly for 1-1/2 hours 4 to 5 times per week will result in more fat loss than exercising every day for 30 minutes. The 30-minute exercise period will use mostly stored muscle and liver glycogen for fuel. Very little fat is involved. On the other hand, the 1-1/2 hour session will use glycogen in the early stages of exercise, then switch to burning fat in the later stages.

There are numerous heart health benefits to exercising in excess of one hour on a regular basis. Triglycerides are used mostly as fat fuel for extended exercise periods. The fatty acid portion of the triglyceride is broken off and sent to the muscles for fuel. When you use triglycerides as fuel, they are taken out of the bloodstream and from fat deposits. Less fats circulating in the blood stream means less fats that can be deposited in the arteries to cause blockages. So, using fat as an exercise fuel can significantly reduce one of the major risks of developing heart disease.

The Role of Protein During Exercise

Protein should play a minor role as an energy source for your exercise sessions. If you do not provide proper carbohydrate stores for exercise, you will break down muscle protein for use as a fuel. Ideally, you should not let this happen. The gains you make in muscle mass will be reversed by the catabolic breakdown of muscle tissue for fuel. The main role of protein in your diet is for growth and repair. The main components of protein are small building blocks called amino acids. The body uses these amino acids to construct and repair cells and tissues. Part of the benefits of exercising is the building of muscle tissue. However, every time we exercise we produce tiny tears in our muscle tissues. It is the job of protein to provide the building blocks for the repair and growth of the muscles we use. The timing of your consumption of proteins can have a significant effect on your exercise performance.

Your main protein consumption should be contained in the meals that follow exercise, not your pre-exercise meal. Your pre-exercise meal should be low in protein for several reasons. Protein, especially animal protein, will remain in your stomach too long to be of any value if consumed only a few hours before exercising. Protein can take up to eight hours to digest. This prolonged digestion period requires water to be diverted from muscles to the intestinal tract in order to aid in digestion.

Protein can take up to eight hours to digest... Eating excess protein can drain you of energy when you most need it...

The process of protein metabolism can leave you dehydrated if you attempt strenuous exercise within a few hours of eating a high-protein meal. Eating excess protein can drain you of energy when you most need it. Protein metabolism is a very time-consuming and energy-draining process. This process involves many chemical reactions and the release of toxic substances such as urea. Your liver and kidneys must work very hard at removing the toxic by-products of protein metabolism. More urine is produced in an effort to eliminate these protein metabolism by-products. Along with the urine, essential minerals such as potassium, calcium, and magnesium are flushed out with the toxic waste products.[6]

Eating excess protein, or eating a high-protein meal too close to exercise time, can significantly dehydrate you and hamper your exercise ability...

The Secrets of Water

I talked about the importance of water in our diet in Chapter 2. Water is the one essential element in our diet that is often overlooked. We are all aware that without it we would be dead in days, yet it is often taken for granted. We drink it when we are thirsty, otherwise we usually don't give it another thought.

The availability of water is critical to energy production. It is for this reason that your exercise ability is greatly influenced by the amount of water available in your body. Whether your goal is to walk a few miles, participate in an aerobics class, or run a marathon, lack of water will hinder your ability to perform.

Most people don't understand the principles of water necessity and utilization. Contrary to popular belief, drinking water when you are thirsty will not provide enough fluid for your body. During exercise, your thirst mechanism is far too deficient a guide to rely on for your water needs. Even after exercise, your thirst mechanism does not accurately indicate your water requirements.

How important is water to your exercise performance? ***A 2-pound water loss can result in a 15% reduction in exercise ability. A 7-pound water loss can hamper your exercise ability up to 30%.***[7] It is easy in hot humid weather to lose 7 pounds of water playing tennis or jogging. If we are losing water rapidly, we could lose 7 pounds of water before our thirst mechanism tells us we are dehydrated. Before I became aware of proper hydration rules, I used to play tennis tournaments severely dehydrated and not even know it. My thirst mechanism didn't even give me a clue as to the state of dehydration I was in.

I have seen and heard many athletes describe their dehydration experiences. In most cases, these athletes didn't even know they were describing dehydration.

Loss of muscle efficiency is one of the first signs to look for in the early stages of dehydration. Other early signs of dehydration include a slow motion sensation or the feeling that you've lost your fine-tuned coordination. Later stages of dehydration can result in a feeling of calm which overcomes you, so that the heat stops bothering you at all, even though it is very hot outside. Your sweat output begins to slow down and change. Your skin becomes more clammy. Other signs are a slight ringing or a clogged sensation in one or both of your ears. I know that when I start to get a ringing sensation in my ears, I'm in big trouble with dehydration.

Until you are aware of the potential dangers of exercising without proper hydration, you are totally oblivious to the signals your body gives you concerning dehydration. Now that you're aware of such potential dangers, you can begin to listen to your body. Look for signs of dehydration in yourself. We all get our own unique dehydration signals. When you discover yours, you will realize they have been there all along, but that you just didn't recognize them.

What is the proper way to hydrate? The first mistake most of us make is to start our exercise session totally or partially dehydrated. Many times, most of us are 20 to 30 minutes into our exercise session before we give water a thought. To compound this mistake, we may not have had a drink for hours before we began exercising. If this sounds like you, then you are substantially handicapping your exercise ability.

The first step to improving your exercise performance is to drink 16 to 20 ounces of fluid 15 to 20 minutes before you begin exercising. The quantity and timing are important for maximum benefit. If you wait until you start exercising, you will be playing "catch up" the whole time you are exercising. This will hamper your success.

The timing of the fluid intake is important because of how your kidneys and bladder function. If you drink your pre-exercise fluid 30 to 45 minutes before exercise, your bladder will be full a few minutes into your exercise session. This is not a big problem if you are just informally practicing and can excuse yourself. However, if you are in a competitive match, you may not be so fortunate.

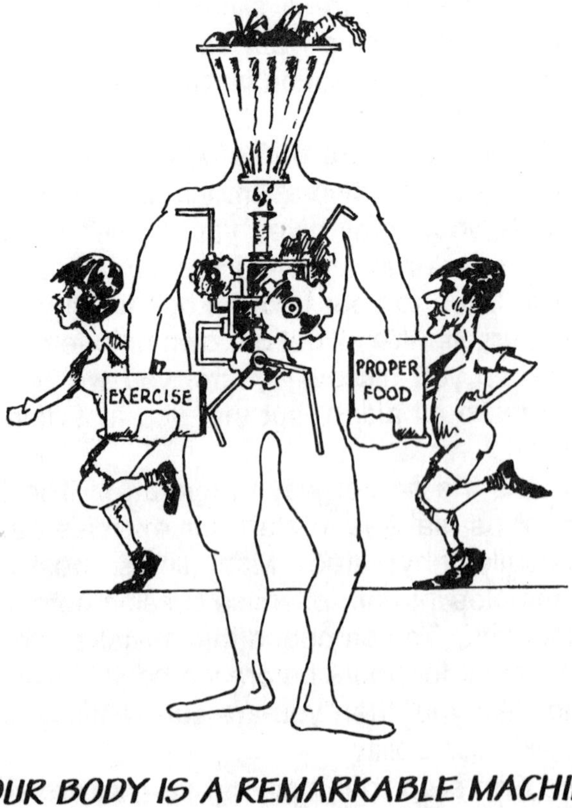

YOUR BODY IS A REMARKABLE MACHINE

When you start to exercise vigorously, raise your heart rate, and breathe rapidly, your body instinctively starts to conserve water. When this happens, your kidneys slow down the production of urine to conserve water for other functions, such as perspiration. Therefore, if you drink your pre-exercise fluid only 15 to 20 minutes before you begin, your bladder should not fill up before the kidneys slow down the production of urine.

Starting your fluid intake after exercise begins will not properly hydrate you since you can only absorb about 1 to 2 pints of fluid an hour from your stomach.[8] If, during a tennis match, you lose 1 gallon of water, while your stomach can only absorb 2 to 4 pints during that period, you will be severely dehydrated and pay dearly for it.

You might say to yourself, "But I don't perspire enough to lose a gallon of water during exercise." The fact is, you may not be aware of how much fluid you are actually losing through perspiration. When you perspire, the water that comes to the surface of your skin evaporates. This evaporation causes a cooling effect on the skin and the blood vessels that are near the surface of the skin. The blood that has been cooled circulates throughout the rest of the body, thus lowering the internal temperature. So you may lose 1 to 2 pints of fluid through evaporation and not even know it. Another way you lose substantial fluid from the body is through breathing. Water is necessary for the breathing process. The lining of the lungs must be kept moist at all times. When you exhale, water is a part of the air you breathe out. The more rapidly you exhale, as in vigorous exercise, the more water you lose.

So you can see that water is lost from the body in many other ways besides just through perspiration or urination. Don't be fooled by the outside temperature. On hot summer days, of course, you will lose the most amount of fluid through perspiration. In the winter, however, you lose more water through exhalation. When the air is cold outside, the body must use water to warm it so that the lungs are not damaged. In the process of moderating the air, warm water from the body is combined with the incoming cool air in an attempt to bring the air closer to body temperature.

Should it be water or sports drinks? This question has long been debated in sports circles. The debate is likely to continue for some time to come. Let's discuss some of the principles of water and mineral absorption which apply to this topic. First of all, as mentioned earlier, about 1 to 2 pints of water per hour can be absorbed from the stomach into the bloodstream during vigorous exercise. If you add substances to the water, such as salt, sugar and minerals, the absorption rate will be less than pure water. For this reason, pure water is the quickest way to hydrate in most circumstances.

During strenuous exercise, however, you do use up carbohydrates for energy production and lose essential minerals through perspiration. If you exercise long enough, you will need to replace them for maximum performance. The question is, should you drink a sports drink like *Gatorade* to replace these lost carbohydrates and minerals, or just plain water? The answer is clear to me. Most commercially-prepared sports drinks will initially do you more harm than good as it pertains to dehydration. Such sports drinks are too concentrated to be absorbed rapidly from the stomach into the bloodstream. These drinks contain more sugar and salt than the body can use. And, as I've already mentioned, the more substances in the water, the slower the absorption rate will be from the stomach to the blood.

If you ever took a chemistry or biology class, you may remember the terms "osmosis" and "active transport." These are the terms which describe how fluids and particles suspended in them, called "solutes," move from one location to another. Simply put, if the fluid in the stomach is of a higher concentration than the blood, the blood will contribute fluid to the stomach to equalize the two solutions.

Where does the fluid needed to balance the two solutions come from? It comes from your muscles and tissues. If the concentration of sugar, salt and minerals from the sports drink is of a higher concentration than the blood, then water from muscles and tissues will be brought to the stomach to reduce the concentration.

You see, the sports drink cannot pass from your stomach into the blood until the two solutions are of relatively equal concentrations. Therefore, in an effort to equalize the concentration of the two solutions, your body will draw water from your muscles to do this. When water is drawn from your muscles during exercise, you will dehydrate even further, thus dramatically reducing muscle efficiency.

In the 1960s, when I was a junior tennis player, the popular wisdom was to take salt tablets to prevent dehydration in the Florida heat. So I faithfully took my quota of salt tablets before I began to play. I couldn't understand why they always had to carry me off the court with cramps associated with dehydration. I now understand that the salt tablets *contributed* to my dehydration rather than preventing it. When the salt tablet hit my stomach, there was a mad rush of water from my muscles and tissues back into the stomach to dilute the salt concentration. Unfortunately, the same principle applies to your *Gatorade* consumption. The concentration of salt, sugar and minerals is greater than your blood, thus causing the flow of water back to the stomach rather than toward your muscles. If you love your sports drink, try diluting it with equals parts of water to lower the concentration of salt, sugar and minerals.

When we exercise heavily, we do need to maintain a proper fluid and electrolyte balance. What is the right concentration of fluids and electrolytes our sports drink should have? The American College of Sports Medicine has determined a useful guideline for maximum concentration of sugar, salt, and potassium in any sports replacement beverage. Every 8-ounce serving of replacement fluid should contain no more than 5.9 grams of sugar, 55 milligrams of sodium, and 46 milligrams of potassium.[9] Most sports drinks on the market today contain significantly greater concentrations of sugar, salt, and minerals.

Fluid and Electrolyte Replacement Guideline
Per 8 Ounces of Fluid

Sugar	5.9 grams
Sodium	55 mg.
Potassium	46 mg.

Adapted from The American College of Sports Medicine

You can buy some sports drinks that have the proper combinations of the necessary carbohydrates and electrolytes. As mentioned earlier, Twin Labs produces two formulations which meet these requirements: *Carboplex* and *Carbo Fuel.* I am sure there are many new sports replacement fluids on the market today that meet the proper requirements. I have no financial interest in the Twin Labs products. I just know they work.

To sum it all up, don't begin exercise dehydrated. Drink 16 to 20 ounces of fluid 15 to 20 minutes before exercise begins. Continue to drink during your exercise period. If you drink a sports drink, make it one with glucose polymers as the carbohydrate source. Also, make sure the concentrations of sugar, salt and electrolytes do not exceed the recommendations of the American College of Sports Medicine. Remember, exercising with a depletion of carbohydrates or water will greatly affect your exercise ability.

POPULAR METHOD

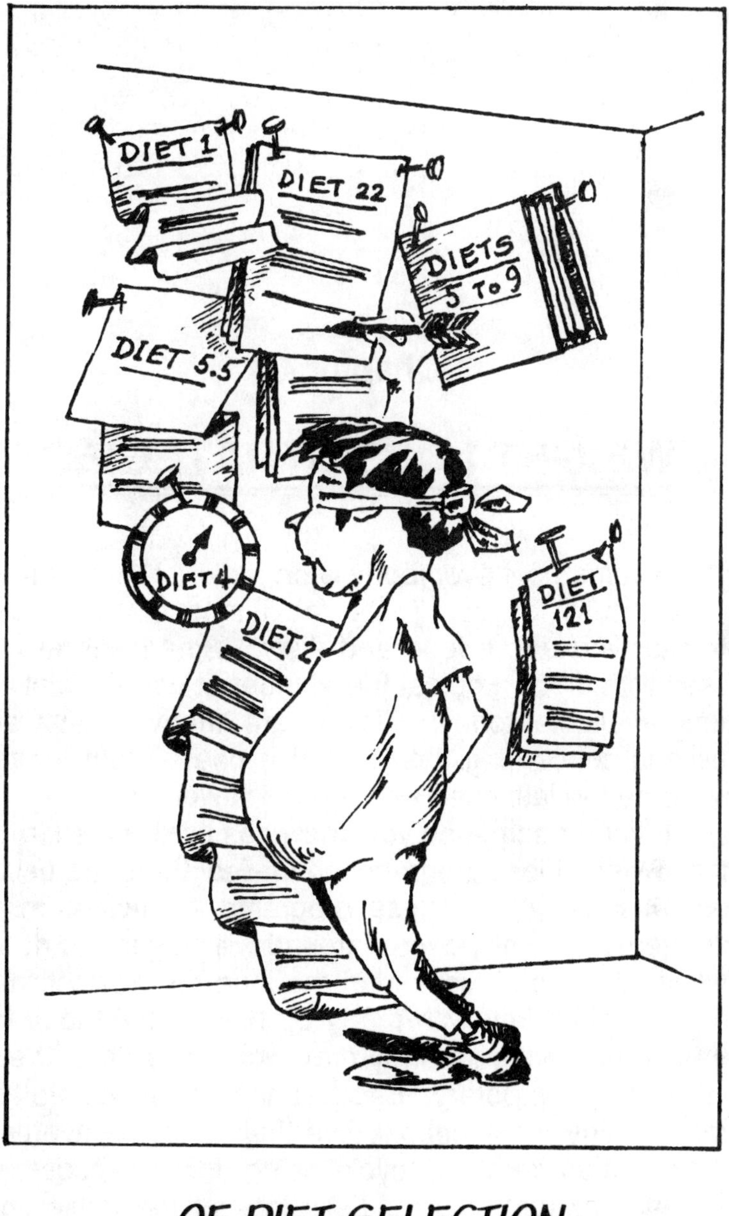

OF DIET SELECTION

Chapter 4

WEIGHT LOSS STRATEGIES

IT seems as if everybody is on a diet. When you turn on the TV, or listen to the radio, most of the commercials are about food and diets. Americans are obsessed with diets. Look at the number of popular diet programs available today! There are many unanswered questions concerning them. Which one is right for me? How come the last one I went on didn't work for long?

If you or someone you know has participated in one of these weight loss programs and failed, there are usually good reasons why. These programs all have common characteristics. They center around will power and denial. Most of us will not succeed in the long run against these odds. The problem with many of these weight loss programs is that, although they may work for a time, the results are only temporary. Because they have worked temporarily, many more people give them a try. Advertising and promotion keep the cycle going: initial success, followed by eventual failure. Let's look at the make-up of some of these weight loss plans.

Popular Weight-Loss Programs

I have talked to many friends and relatives who have participated in popular diet programs such as *Weight Watchers* or *Nutri-Systems.* The results have all been much the same. They all got excited about making a commitment to a new program, then followed it religiously for a few months or even a year.

In time, however, the newness and the commitment begin to fade. Once your resolve fades, the diet plan is doomed. These plans are not necessarily bad diet plans. Most of them work, to an extent, as long as your will power is intact. But I know of no one who has been able to stay on any of these plans for a good portion of their lives. They all take pounds off and then put pounds back on again.

Calorie-Restricted Diets

After you fail to keep the pounds off because you no longer have the will power to stay on one of these diets, you decide to starve the pounds off. Many of you have already tried this route. Don't do it. It doesn't work. Your body will fight you on this one.

Let me explain how your body reacts to a low calorie diet. Everybody has their own rate of burning calories. We're similar to automobiles in this respect. A car has a certain rate at which it burns fuel, usually expressed in miles per gallon (mpg). Every function of our body requires fuel. If you want your car to drive, you have to put fuel in the tank. The food we eat is converted into this fuel. Unlike cars, however, our bodies can adjust the amount of fuel they burn. It is this ability to adjust fuel burned which guarantees that your low-calorie diet will ultimately fail.

The rate at which you burn calories while inactive is called your *basal metabolic rate* (BMR). Let's say your BMR is 60 calories per hour while you are resting. When you go on a calorie-restricted diet of 600 - 900 calories per day, your body thinks you are starving. Your remarkable body has the ability to change the rate at which you burn calories in an effort to protect your life. Your rate of burning calories could go down to 30 - 40 calories per hour, instead of your normal 60. What do you think this does to your weight-loss plans? Well, you will still shed pounds, but it won't seem as though you are losing them in proportion to the amount of calories you are eliminating.

The worst is yet to come. It wouldn't be so bad if the only problem with a low-calorie diet was the speed of weight loss. The main problem with this type of diet has to do with the re-calibrating of your metabolic rate (the rate at which you burn calories). Eventually, if you are persistent, you can reach your desired weight by starving the pounds off. You begin to relax. You decide to return to a normal diet to maintain your weight loss. The only problem is that your body won't re-calibrate your metabolism just because you want it to. It may be 6 months or more before your rate of burning calories returns to normal. During this 6-month period, you gain all the lost weight back, and then some. I have spoken to countless numbers of people who nod their heads when I describe this chain of events. They have all tried this method of weight loss and failed.

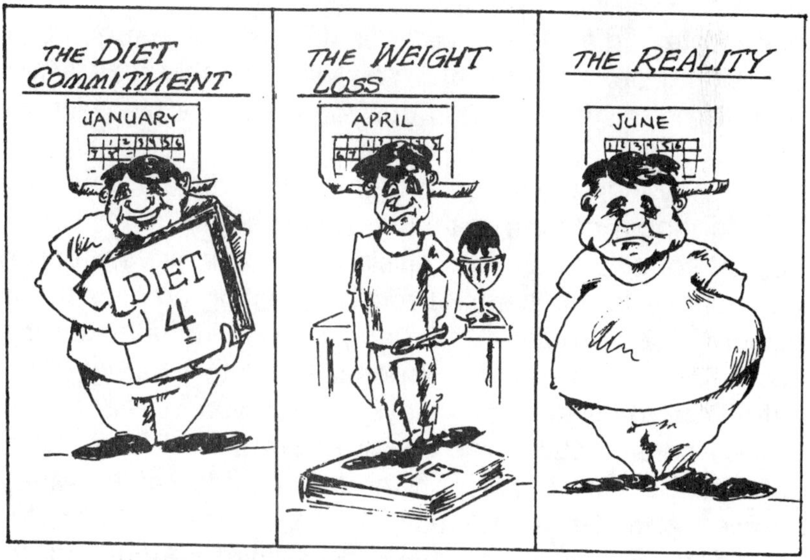

"Yo-Yo dieting" is the term used to describe losing weight and then rapidly gaining it back again. This type of dieting complicates your ability to lose weight in the future. Each time you re-calibrate your metabolism down to burn less calories per hour by reducing your caloric intake, it takes longer and longer to return to normal after you stop the calorie restrictions. After you repeat this cycle a number of times, your body will form a "set-point" concerning calories burned per hour. Your metabolism will resist any attempt to change this rate of burning. Many of you who have dieted repeatedly are already experiencing this phenomenon. If a low-calorie diet sounds appealing to you, don't fall into the "yo-yo" trap. You may alter your metabolism for a long time to come.

High-Protein Diets

High-protein diets are another group of fad diets which are less than optimal. Here again, these types of diets will give you initial success. The main theory behind high-protein diets is that calories are lost in the process of converting protein into fat. You will probably lose a few pounds on this type of diet, but you will pay a big price for them.

Anyone staying on a high-protein diet for any extended length of time is taking a high health risk. Under normal conditions, the processing of protein is very taxing on systems in the body. Protein digestion creates many poisonous by-products that have to be eliminated by the body. The main organs responsible for this heavy elimination are the liver and kidneys. When you increase your protein consumption well beyond normal needs, you put an overwhelming burden on the liver and kidneys. Many people who have stayed on high-protein diets for extended periods of time have developed serious kidney problems. You can permanently damage your kidneys on a high-protein diet. The dialysis business has profited well from these types of diets.

While watching the news on TV the other day, I noticed a segment about the health of one of the actors in the popular TV show, *Knots Landing*. He had developed complete kidney failure. Toxic waste was backing up into his stomach because his kidneys ceased to function. He was rushed to the hospital and immediately put on a dialysis machine. The doctors said he was one of the lucky ones to have survived. His physicians indicated that the main cause of his kidney failure was due to the high-protein diet he had been on in an effort to lose weight. I don't think it was worth the price.

The Lifetime Diet

Now here's the good news! There *is* a diet that's perfect for you. It has none of the problems all those other popular diets have. It's not low-calorie and it's not high-protein. You'll also be happy to know that with this diet you'll never have to count calories or go hungry again! You'll even be able to stop the vicious "yo-yo" cycles you have probably experienced before. In fact, this diet is the only way you can ever break the "yo-yo" cycle.

"...with this diet, you'll never have to count calories or go hungry again!"

I'll call this diet the "Lifetime Diet" because it's the last diet you will ever need. I know, I know. I can just see you shaking your head and saying, "I've heard that one before!" But read on. By the time I finish describing this diet, you'll have to agree with me. Not only is this diet great for weight loss, but it's also the diet of choice for maximum life span. Let's look at some of the principals of this diet.

Calories don't count. Most diets don't work because of the hunger factor. Sooner or later, if you stay on a diet that emphasizes set amounts of calories or portions, you will fail. The Lifetime Diet has no calorie or portion restrictions. On this diet, when you're hungry, you simply eat. It's as simple as that! Of course, you must eat the *right kinds* of foods, but the quantities are never restricted.

Low protein is the way to go. A high-protein diet will destroy your kidneys, tax your liver to its limits, and increase the overall burden on your digestive system. The Lifetime Diet is based on a low-protein diet. The typical American diet consists of 3 times the quantity of protein needed for optimal health. The Lifetime Diet protein guidelines are based on the National Academy of Sciences' Recommended Dietary Allowances (RDA). The

RDA for protein in adult females and males is 44 and 56 grams respectively. The RDA for protein has a safety margin built in it, so you needn't worry about consuming too little protein if you follow the guideline. It doesn't take a very large portion of protein-rich food to meet your requirements, so go easy on this type of food.

Fat should be 10 - 15% of your calories. Controlling your daily fat intake is the heart of the Lifetime Diet. Fat grams are the only thing you will ever need to count again in your diet.

In order to learn how to recognize and count fat grams, write down all the foods you eat for a 2-week period. Then look up the fat gram content of these foods on the tables I have provided for you at the back of this book. After you do this for 2 weeks, you will have memorized the fat gram content of your favorite foods. If you love pizza, for example, you'll soon learn that 2 slices of a medium thin and crispy *Pizza Hut* pizza has 17 grams of fat. When I splurge and have this kind of pizza, I know that I have to be careful with my fat gram intake the rest of the day.

Often times our perception of what we are doing is nowhere near reality. This is often the case when it comes to the food we eat. Most Americans consume 2 to 3 times the maximum quantity of fat that they should and don't even realize it. If I could help you make only one lifestyle change in order to lose weight and improve your health, it would be to reduce the quantity of fat in your diet. Excess dietary fat is the main villain I have exposed to you throughout this book. Control your fat habit, and you will be on your way to success in weight loss and improved health.

Below is a formula for converting fat grams and calories into the percentage of "fat calories" you consume in your diet.

Fat Gram Conversion Guidelines

- Using the food charts at the back of this book, count the number of fat grams in the foods you have eaten.
- Each gram of fat has 9 calories.
- Multiply your total fat grams by 9 to determine the number of fat calories you have consumed.
- Divide your fat calories by your total calories to get the percentage of calories from fat.

For example, if you consume 2000 calories per day and your fat grams are 60, you would multiply 60 grams of fat by 9 calories per gram, to get a total of 540 fat calories. You would then divide 540 by 2000 to get a decimal answer of .27 (multiply .27 x 100 = 27%), which represents the percentage of calories from fat in your diet.

If all that fancy math wears you out, a simple rule of thumb is to keep your fat grams between 20 - 40 per day, depending on the number of calories you consume. If you are eating around 1500 calories a day, then 20 grams of fat will keep you well within your optimal intake. On the other hand, if you are eating close to 3000 calories per day, then your target fat grams should be around 40 grams.

High-complex carbohydrates are the answer. Maybe you're saying, "Okay, so I can't have a high-protein diet, and I can't have a high-fat diet. Well, just what am I supposed to eat?" I'll tell you what you're supposed to eat -- just what you were designed to eat: high-fiber complex carbohydrates! And here's the good news: you can eat as much of them as you want!

Carbohydrates are the most misunderstood food group in our diets.

Some common misconceptions about carbohydrates:

- they will make you fat
- they're harmful for diabetics
- they have too many calories.

All of these beliefs are wrong. High-fiber complex carbohydrates are the least likely food to make you gain weight. Carbohydrates have the primary function of providing immediate fuel for many chemical reactions going on inside the body. Your body was designed to utilize carbohydrates for everything else before it stores them as fat. In order for carbohydrates to be stored as fat, they must first be converted into a form that can be stored as fat. The process of converting these carbohydrates is very wasteful. If the conversion is made, there are fewer calories left to be stored as fat.

If you add lots of fiber to the carbohydrates, then even less of the calories you have eaten are absorbed into the blood from the intestinal tract. Fiber has the tendency to interfere with the absorption of calories by binding them up in its mesh-like structure and carrying them out of the body unabsorbed. Fiber also slows down the absorption of carbohydrates into the blood, thus aiding the diabetic condition rather than harming it. Another great benefit to eating high-fiber foods is that they make you feel full in a hurry. It's hard to overeat on a high-fiber diet.

On the other hand, it is extremely efficient for your body to store dietary fat as excess body fat. The main function of fat is to provide storage of energy for future use. In times of famine, we would be grateful for this energy reserve. Unfortunately for most of us, our storage tanks are full and there is no famine in sight. Unlike carbohydrates, dietary fat needs no conversion to be stored as fat. Therefore, it is very efficient for your dietary fat to be stored as body fat. This is the main reason counting calories doesn't work. All calories are not created equal in their use in the body.

All calories are not created equal...

During one of my lectures in a pre-med anatomy class at Pasco Hernando Community College, I was discussing nutrition and metabolism when the topic of weight loss diets surfaced. It seems that every time food is discussed in a group setting, weight loss diets are always the hottest topic. Question after question came up about which type of diet is the best, and which is the best way to lose weight. I told the students that weight loss was simple. All you had to do was eat *more* food, not less. This statement drew a lot of blank stares. "How can we eat more and lose weight?" the students asked.

When you eat more of the *right foods*, I told them, your metabolism will be accelerated to burn more calories. If you eat a high-calorie, high-fat diet, your metabolism will slow down and store more calories.

Just when I was really getting into this discussion with the class, one of the students raised his hand and said, "I know just what you mean." I gave him a nod to encourage him to go on. He then told us how he had gone on a high-calorie, high-complex carbohydrate, low-fat diet, consuming about 3200 calories a day. His diet consisted of large quantities of raw vegetables, fruits and grains. In spite of the large amount of calories consumed, he lost 30 pounds in 3 months and never felt better. He said that his energy levels had never been higher than they were while on this diet, and he felt as though he could do anything. It was a perfect example of the point I was trying to make. It was such a perfect testimony, in fact, that I wondered if people might think I'd arranged the whole thing.

But then the man said, "Wait. There's more to my story."

I let him continue.

He told us that he later went to his doctor for a routine physical and decided to share the great news about his diet with him. Upon hearing about all the extra food he was eating, his doctor was alarmed. He told him to get off the diet immediately, that it had too many calories. All that food couldn't possibly be healthy, he told him. So the doctor convinced his patient to return to a so-called "normal" diet. The student went home discouraged, but decided to listen to his doctor and return to the diet he recommended. He reduced his calories down to about 2500 a day, plus chucked a lot of the high-complex carbohydrates he'd been eating, and returned to a "normal" 40% fat level diet. Within a few months he gained all his weight back and then some.

I was angry, though not surprised, that a medical doctor could give such erroneous advice. But this doctor's advice was typical of so many in the medical profession who are nutritionally uneducated. Just because a physician knows a great deal about surgical procedures does not guarantee that he necessarily knows everything there is to know about nutrition.

Needless to say, after our lecture, this student went back on his high-fiber, high-complex carbohydrate, low-fat diet with new conviction and fervor. I am sure that he will be able to repeat his past weight loss performance, even if he consumes 3200 calories a day. The moral of the story is: calories don't count. It's not *how many* calories you eat, but *what kind* of calories they are that counts.

The Lifetime Diet Summary

The Lifetime Diet is built on the foundation of high-fiber complex carbohydrates. Your main sources of these types of foods should be fruits, vegetables, whole grains and a small amount of nuts and seeds. For those of you who are not convinced that vegetarianism is the way to go, a small amount of lean meat and fish can be eaten. If you really want to reach "super health," however, you will have to make animal products a very small part of your overall diet.

Cut your fat intake to the desirable range of 10 - 15% of your diet. Don't worry about where you are going to get your protein. if you eat according to my food plan, It's almost impossible to be deficient in protein. The only way to come up short in the protein department is if you are eating an extremely low-calorie diet. If you are eating too few calories, then you will be deficient in many nutrients. Contrary to popular belief, there is protein in just about everything we eat. Even fruits and vegetables have protein in them. It is these small amounts of protein that can easily add up to your RDA of protein without worrying about needing a piece of meat to fulfill your requirements. When you are hungry, eat freely from the wide range of fruits, vegetables and whole grains available, including potatoes, rice, and pastas. Make sure you eat whole, unrefined foods whenever possible. White refined bread and flour are not high-fiber complex carbohydrates. They are only the shells left after just about everything beneficial in them has been stripped away. Whole grain breads, brown rice, and baked potatoes with the skin are high-fiber complex carbohydrates.

The only trouble you will get into with the high-fiber complex carbohydrates is what you cook them with or put on them after cooking them, such as sauces or dressings. Try to eat as many of your fruits and vegetables raw.

Cooking destroys some nutrients and enzymes that are beneficial to maximum health.

Don't count calories and never go hungry again.

Eat small, frequent meals if you are hungry. Your body handles small, frequent meals much better than one or two large meals. Eat after you have exercised. The calories you eat immediately after exercise will be used first to restore your muscle and liver glycogen levels. These are the places where stored calories were used up during exercise. Your body is a remarkable machine. Feed it right and it will reward you with boundless energy and remarkably good health.

DON'T COUNT CALORIES

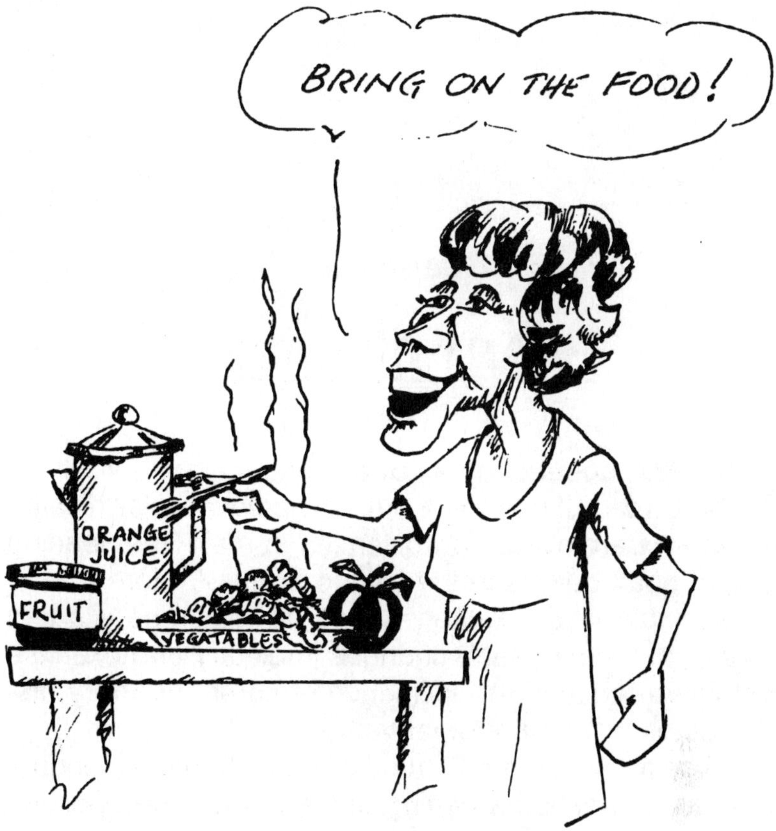

AND NEVER GO HUNGRY AGAIN

Chapter 5

HEART DISEASE

IN 1982, about one-half of all deaths among adults in the United States were due to cardiovascular diseases.[1] Cardiovascular diseases remain the leading cause of adult deaths in the United States.[2] More than 5 million people in the United States have coronary artery disease. In recent years, changes in dietary and exercise habits have reduced the incidence of coronary artery disease deaths by about 2% per year.

The most common cause of heart disease in industrialized countries is hardening of the arteries (arteriosclerosis) and fatty deposits in the arteries. Hardening, or thickening, of the arteries is caused by the accumulation of fatty deposits inside the arterial wall. The problem results when we eat too much animal and dairy fat (including milk and cheese). Excess circulating fats in the blood stream (imagine a load of twinkies in the blood stream!) enlarge and clump together in the form of fatty deposits which, since they're too chubby to get thru or go far, attach themselves to the insides of the arterial walls (lazy bums!). This process begins to narrow the arterial opening, which results in increased pressure of the blood against the arterial wall.

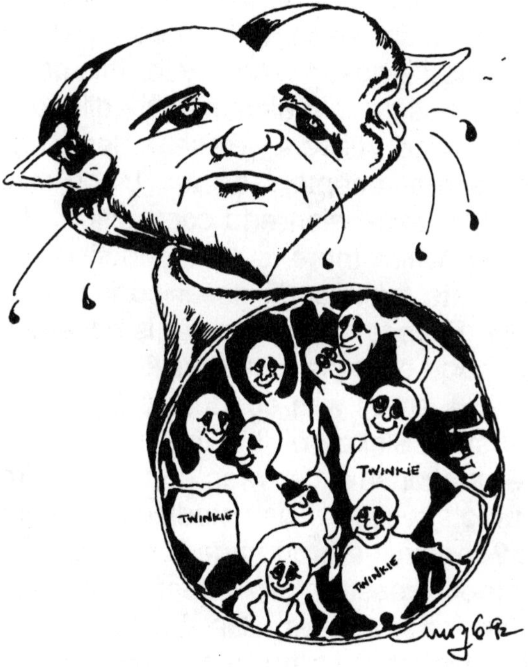

Normally, the walls of the arteries are very flexible and elastic like a new rubber hose, expanding and contracting with each heartbeat. The buildup of fatty plaques on the arterial walls causes the arterial wall to lose some of its elasticity, much as would a garden hose left out in the sun. The more rigid the arterial walls become, the greater the resistance to blood flow, resulting in an increased workload for the heart.

High Blood Pressure and Sodium

Many of us have been warned in recent years about the harmful effects of excessive salt in our diets. Excess salt contributes to an increase in blood pressure. Although it is not yet clear which mechanism causes our blood pressure to increase with added salt, recent research has yielded a possible theory for this phenomenon. Normal blood pressure is maintained by dilation and constriction of the blood vessels. Researchers have discovered that there are receptors on the blood vessel walls which control this expansion and contraction. High blood pressure results when there is a malfunction in these receptors which lets the blood vessel contract but not expand properly. Excess salt in the diet is believed to play a part in the damage of these receptors.[3]

In 1989, a study was conducted by Ross D. Feldman and Christine Sinkey of the University of Iowa to investigate the relationship between sodium intake and the elasticity of blood vessels. They studied a group of people aged 48 to 72, against a group aged 20 to 31, all of whom had normal blood pressure. Volunteers in both groups ate a high-salt diet for four days. On the fifth day, scientists injected each subject in both groups with a small amount of a drug which causes blood vessels to constrict. A small dose of isoproterenol, an adrenaline-like substance which causes dilation, was also administered. They found that blood vessels in the older group dilated only half as much as those in the younger group.[4]

After the researchers gave both groups a low-salt diet for four days, the blood vessels of the older subjects dilated as much as those of the younger subjects. These results suggest that older people can stave off an age-associated malfunction in their blood vessel receptors and reduce their risk of hypertension by reducing dietary salt.[5]

It is believed that excess salt in the diet can damage arterial walls without even increasing a person's blood pressure. The salt is believed to scar the interior arterial walls, thus leaving lesions on which circulating blood fats can attach. This process begins to explain how coronary artery diseases and high blood pressure intertwine.

The Infamous Cholesterol Connection

No discussion of heart disease can be complete without mentioning the cholesterol connection. What is cholesterol anyway? Cholesterol is a sterol, a member of the fat family. When we speak of fats we are really talking about lipids. Lipids include triglycerides, phospholipids, and sterols. So we can see that cholesterol is a fat.

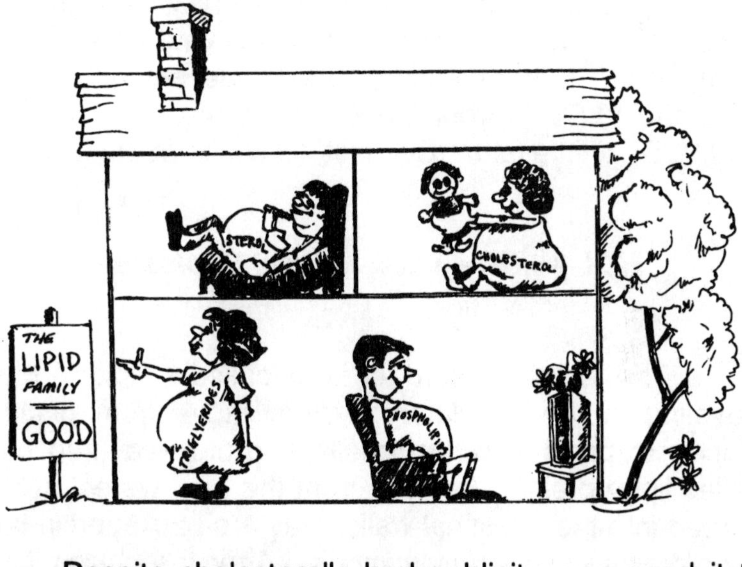

Despite cholesterol's bad publicity, you need it to survive. Let's look at some of its roles. Cholesterol is manufactured by the liver and converted into hormones, such as the sex and adrenal hormones. Cholesterol is also used in the formation of bile acids which are excreted from the bile ducts into the intestines to emulsify fats during the digestive process. Isn't it ironic? Without cholesterol you couldn't even digest fat. Cholesterol is also packaged with lipoproteins for transport in the blood to cells that need lipids. The cholesterol is used by the cells to form their outer membrane. It is estimated that more than nine-tenths of the body's cholesterol is located in the cell's membranes.[6] So you can see that cholesterol plays a very important part in your life.

Let's talk a little about the different components which make up the thing we call cholesterol. Cholesterol isn't just one component, but a group of different components. HDL (High Density Lipoprotein), LDL (Low Density Lipoprotein), and VLDL (Very Low Density Lipoprotein) are all components of "total cholesterol." They are formed in the packaging of cholesterol with lipoproteins. Hence, the term we know as "cholesterol" actually includes these lipoproteins. So, in order to calculate your Total Cholesterol Count, it is necessary to add the amount of HDL, LDL and VLDL in your blood. We'll discuss HDL, LDL, and VLDL a little later. But, first, let's look at the fats.

HDL + LDL + VLDL = Total Cholesterol

The technical word for fat is called a "lipid." Lipids traveling in the circulatory system move from place to place, wrapped in water-repellent, protein-covered coats called lipoproteins. As lipids from the food we eat are absorbed into the intestinal walls, they are packaged in large lipoproteins called *chylomicrons*. After the chylomicrons are released from the intestines, they travel through the circulatory system to all the cells of the body, allowing the cells to pick up lipids as needed. Lipids which originate from the processing of fat in the liver are called *very low density lipoproteins* (VLDLs). These lipids are composed of triglycerides, cholesterol, phospholipids, and proteins which are then transported to other parts of the body for use. As the different cells around the body remove triglycerides from the VLDL, *low density lipoproteins* (LDLs) are formed. The liver and intestines also manufacture another kind of lipoprotein called *high density lipoprotein* (HDL). HDLs appear to have the function of transporting unused cholesterol back to the liver for reuse or elimination.

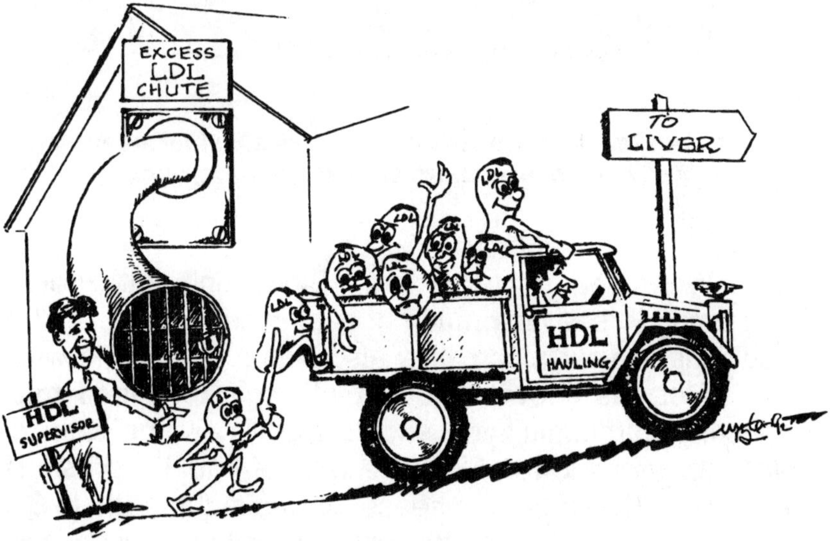

Don't judge fat too harshly. Fat serves many important purposes in the body. Fat insulates against temperature extremes and protects the vital organs from shocks. It provides an energy supply and is also responsible for transporting the fat soluble vitamins. So, we need to realize that, without fat on our bodies and in our diet, life would not be possible. It is the ***excess*** fats we must decrease in order to achieve longevity.

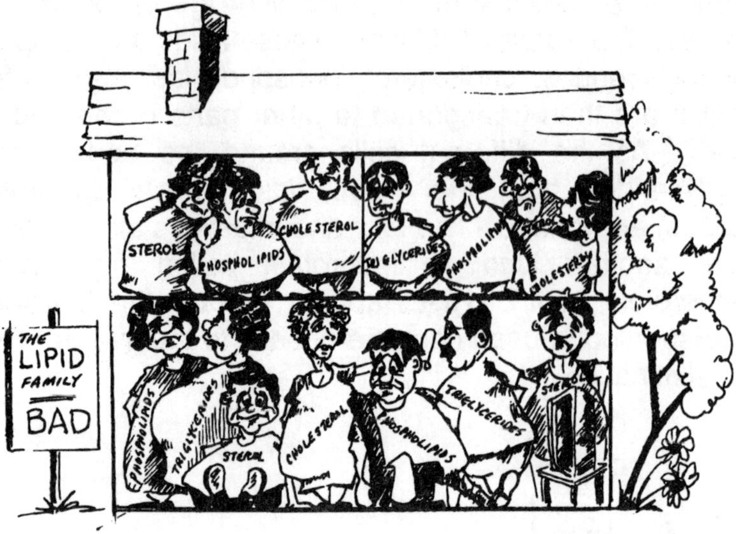

It's not the existence of fats in our system that's bad - it's when they overcrowd that we're in trouble.

When your doctor orders a Blood Lipid (fat) Profile, he is trying to see how much of each type of blood lipid is circulating in your blood. He also wants to know in what ratio. Besides knowing your total cholesterol and total triglyceride amounts, you should also know the ratio of *total cholesterol* to *total HDL*. A ratio of 5 to 1 represents an average risk of heart disease. Improve that ratio to 3.5 to 1 and you will have cut your risk of heart disease in half. As part of your personal program for longevity, you should know your Blood Lipid Profile and ratio of Total Cholesterol to HDL.

Table 5.1 outlines some blood cholesterol numbers and their interrelationships. In our earlier discussions regarding cholesterol, HDL, and LDL, I indicated that HDL and LDL are components of total cholesterol. **HDL** is considered the **"good cholesterol"** because its main function

TABLE 5.1
HEART HEALTH NUMBERS

TYPE OF CHOLESTEROL	DESIRABLE	UNDESIRABLE
Total Cholesterol	150	>180
Ratio Total Chol/HDL	3/1	>5/1
HDL Cholesterol	>70	<35
LDL	<100	>160

The ">" symbol means greater than.
The "<" symbol means less than.
The unit of measure is mg/100ml (for example 150 mg of cholesterol per 100ml of blood.)

is to escort excess cholesterol back to the liver for reprocessing or elimination. HDL's role as an eliminator of excess circulating cholesterol makes it beneficial for you to have a somewhat high proportion of HDL to total cholesterol, as suggested in the following table.

The numbers in the "DESIRABLE" column represent a very low risk of heart disease. Although these numbers are more stringent than orthodox medical advice at this time, longevity studies indicate that the numbers in the desirable column are the ones you need to strive for if you are to have a chance at maximum life span.

Before leaving this section, I'll need to throw a little gasoline on the fire, just to remind you that everything doesn't always fit into neat little packages. Many of us have been told to keep our weight under control as one means to protect ourselves from heart disease and cancer. Weight control is indeed a very effective way to aid in the control of these diseases. However, the twist is that, if you go on a weight loss program, your blood fats may begin to elevate during the process of losing weight. A recent research study highlights this finding.

Nutrition researcher, Stephen Phinney, of the University of California, has conducted a study on the blood cholesterol levels of overweight men and women on diets. He discovered that, as the participants lost weight, their blood cholesterol levels initially dropped. After approximately four months on calorie-restricted diets, blood cholesterol levels began to rise, on the average, 10 to 30 milligrams per deciliter. "We suspected," says Phinney, "that, as fat cells shrink, the cholesterol stored inside them is forced into the blood." To confirm this, he took tiny samples of fat tissue from 6 other overweight women before, during, and after weight loss. As predicted, cholesterol levels fell in the women's body fat stores during the diet, but rose in their blood.[7] A doctor's first response to an elevated Blood Lipid Profile is to put the patient on a restrictive diet. After a period of time to see how the patient responds to such a diet, the physician will do a follow-up blood lipid study. If there is no significant improvement, the doctor may prescribe cholesterol-lowering drugs.

As we have just learned from the preceding study, your cholesterol level may rise for a period, then begin to drop as expected. If your doctor does your follow-up Blood Lipid Profile while the fat cells are shrinking and squeezing the cholesterol out into the blood, the test will show misleading information. Your doctor may then prescribe unnecessary drug therapy for you. It's important for you to understand that your weight needs to be stable for a few months before you can get an accurate Blood Lipid Profile.

The moral of the story is: *educate yourself.* This does not mean you should ignore your doctor's advice.

Your doctor is highly trained and dedicated to the promotion of your health. But no one person knows it all. You must take some personal responsibility for your own well being.

In summary, the important information you need to know about blood fats is that: (1) Low density lipoproteins (LDLs) are the fats from your diet and those manufactured from the liver and intestines which travel to the cells to be used in their many functions. (2) High density lipoproteins (HDLs) are the fats manufactured from the liver and intestines whose function is to accumulate and transport excess cholesterol back to the liver for reuse. We need both forms of fats. As we mentioned previously, the HDLs go around accumulating as much of the excess blood fats as they can and transport them back to the liver. Since most of us eat much more fat than necessary, it is beneficial for us to maintain a somewhat high quantity of HDLs circulating in the blood to handle this excess fat.

What is the Main Cause of Heart Disease?

The main cause of heart disease (the Number One killer in most industrialized countries of the world) is due to what we put into our mouths. To be more specific, the largest cause involves the ***amount*** and ***type*** of fat we consume. Other major contributing factors include excess salt intake and smoking. Many people find it hard to believe that most cases of heart disease can have these simple causes. Let me tell you a story that emphasizes this point.

One afternoon, while lecturing in a college anatomy class on nutrition and metabolism, the subject of diet and heart disease came up. We were discussing the effects of excess dietary fat and the development of arterial blockages. I had mentioned that excess dietary fat would not only add extra pounds to your body, but would also use the extra fat to clog your arteries. A student raised her hand at this point in the discussion and asked a question. "I'm lucky," she said. "I eat a lot of high-fat junk food, including hotdogs, chips and candybars, and I never gain any weight. My body must not store very much fat. Does this mean, since I'm thin, I don't clog my arteries either?"

In response, I told her the following story about a man named Lou.

Lou is an outdoors kind of guy in his 40s. His daytime job is in maintenance. A typical work day for Lou might include digging a ditch for an hour or two, painting buildings, or hauling lumber. So you can see that he is not sedentary, but leads an active lifestyle. He has a thin, trim build and looks like a man in good physical condition. He is probably about 5'9" tall and weighs between 130-140 pounds. This is an ideal weight for a man of this height. Lou came over to talk to me one afternoon, hearing that I was just finishing a book on health and fitness. He wanted all the information I had on heart disease. You see, Lou was recovering from triple by-pass heart surgery. Naturally, he wanted to do whatever was in his power to prevent his having to go through that procedure again. He had become an avid student of heart disease and its prevention.

Lou's story is not an uncommon scenario. Having a lean frame and an active lifestyle does not necessarily protect you from heart disease. Just because someone doesn't look fat on the outside doesn't mean they don't have fat on the inside. If you eat a high-fat diet, you will clog your arteries. It is a very rare person who can escape this fact. Lou was very unaware of this connection. Judging by Lou's strong thirst for knowledge on the subject, I doubt that he will fall into this trap again.

When we talk about fats in the diet, we are mostly talking about *triglycerides* since they are the most abundant type. Triglycerides come in many shapes and sizes, but they are all composed of a glycerol molecule and three fatty acids. The three fatty acids are the "tri' in the term *triglyceride.* The glycerol portion of the triglyceride is always the same, but the fatty acids may vary in length and degree of saturation. It is the degree of saturation which is of concern to us regarding its connection to heart disease. Now let's look at several classifications regarding the degree of fatty acid saturation.

Saturated Fats

A fatty acid is an organic molecule that contains a long chain of carbon atoms with hydrogen atoms bonded to most or all the carbons. If the triglyceride is a saturated fat, then each carbon atom is bonded to two hydrogen atoms. If every carbon atom in the chain is bonded with two hydrogen atoms, then the chain is said to be saturated with all the hydrogens it can possibly hold. Scientific studies have shown a definite correlation between a diet high in these saturated fats and heart disease.

How can we identify these saturated fats? Simple! Every carbon has two hydrogen atoms attached to it. Saturated fats are solid, straight molecules that can pack tightly together, creating a fat that is solid at room temperature. Can you identify some of these types? Sure! They are the animal fats, such as butter and lard. You may want to think of it like this:

saturated = tightly packed/solid(ie, butter/lard)

These are the fats that have been suggested in elevated blood cholesterol levels and in unfavorable ratios of HDLs to LDLs. Studies have indicated that these fats cause us the most health problems by clogging arteries.

Unsaturated Fats

In unsaturated fats, the carbon atoms do not all have hydrogen atoms bonded to them. In unsaturated fats, one or more of the carbons may be missing hydrogens. In nature, carbon atoms must contain four bonds. In order to satisfy the natural order of things, two of the carbons in the chain can form double bonds with each other. Thus, you are left with gaps in the hydrogen chain. Now a chain of carbons with one double carbon bond is called a *monounsaturated fat*. A chain with two or more double carbon bonds is called a *polyunsaturated fat*. How can we identify the unsaturated fats? This is not a difficult task either. Because there are missing hydrogen bonds in an unsaturated fat, it is not as rigid as a saturated fat. An unsaturated fat is flimsy at room temperature. Therefore, we can describe an unsaturated fat as liquid at room temperature. An example of unsaturated fats is vegetable oil.

unsaturated = liquid at room temperature
(ie, vegetable oil)

Studies have indicated that these fats are more desirable in our diets because they have less artery clogging ability and more favorably affect our ratios of HDL (the good cholesterol) to LDL (the bad cholesterol).

Hydrogenated Fats

Now that we have grasped the meaning of a saturated fat (a fat which has all the carbon atoms bonded with hydrogen atoms to form a stiff, solid fat, such as butter or lard), and the unsaturated fats (fats with one or more hydrogen bonds missing, thus making them more liquid at room temperature -- generally from vegetable sources such as vegetable oils), we can now explore the mystery of h*ydrogenated fats.*

What is a hydrogenated fat? Is a hydrogenated fat saturated or unsaturated?

A hydrogenated fat is usually derived from a plant source, which would indicate that it is unsaturated. But a hydrogenated fat is created by adding hydrogen bonds to an unsaturated fat, thus making it partially or totally saturated. When an unsaturated fat is hydrogenated, most of the beneficial qualities that were present in the unsaturated fat are eliminated. In the opinion of many scientists, a hydrogenated fat acts like a saturated fat in the blood. As if that were not enough, there is another twist to the hydrogenated fat story. The process of adding hydrogen bonds to an unsaturated fat creates an unnatural type of fat called a t*rans fat.* These trans fats have unnatural types of bonds which have unnatural effects in the blood. Studies have indicated that these unnatural fats adversely effect our cholesterol levels in the blood.

hydrogenated = altered fat
(ie, margarine, peanut butter, salad dressing)

One such study performed by Ronald B. Mensink and Martin B. Katan of Agricultural University in Wageningen, The Netherlands, shows that the process of hydrogenating unsaturated fats restructures unsaturated fats into trans fats. This altered fat produces blood cholesterol changes that are equal to or, in some cases, worse than saturated fats.[8]

How do we identify hydrogenated fats? The answer is tricky. The more hydrogen bonds that are filled in the unsaturated fat, the more solid at room temperature the hydrogenated fat will be. This also applies to the degree of saturation of the new fat. Here we have some light at the end of the tunnel. The harder a hydrogenated fat is at room temperature, the more saturated a fat it is. Therefore, the converse is also true. The softer a hydrogenated fat is at room temperature, the more unsaturated it is. When consuming hydrogenated fats, a typical example is margarine. Try to use the ones that are more liquid at room temperature. The squeeze bottles of margarine, and even the tubs of margarine, are less hydrogenated than the stick margarines. In this way, you will be limiting your exposure to the "trans fats."

Two other examples of hydrogenated food products commonly eaten are commercially prepared peanut butter and many salad dressings. To be sure, read the labels of food products for the term "hydrogenated" in the list of ingredients.

What Can We Do to Prevent Heart Disease?

We have discussed some causes of heart disease. Now we must talk about what can be done to prevent it. Heart disease develops not as a result of any single factor. It develops as a result of many interrelated risk factors combining to cause damage to the blood vessels or the heart muscle itself. There are, however, several very powerful risk factors which cause a great percentage of damage to the heart.

Smoking

One of the most powerful risk factors contributing to heart disease is smoking. Experts agree that, in order to reduce heart disease risk, it is essential to quit cigarette smoking. Dr. Norman Kaplan, of the University of Texas Southwestern Medical School, says that, in order to reverse heart disease, "the first and most important of all is to quit smoking. There's nothing you can do that will improve your health status quicker than quitting smoking."[9]

University of Minnesota cardiologist, Arthur Leon, agrees. "You get the biggest bang for your buck by not smoking," he says. "Most of the sudden deaths from a coronary event occur in people who are smokers. For those who have already had one heart attack, it is doubly important."[10] If you don't smoke, great! If you do smoke, you must quit if you are to have a chance at longevity.

Fat Consumption

Apart from smoking, the next biggest factor, and the one that is, for the most part, in your control, is the monitoring and control of your blood lipids. Notice that I didn't say, "the monitoring and control of your cholesterol." Your Total Blood Cholesterol Level is only one factor that comprises your Blood Lipid Profile. You also need to know about your triglyceride, HDL and LDL levels, along with your ratio of Total Cholesterol to HDL. In order to keep your Blood Lipid Profile looking like the ideal numbers listed in *Table 5.1*, you must have a diet that is considerably lower in fat than the one recommended by The American Heart Association. A diet containing 30% of its total calories from fat, which is the recommendation of The American Heart Association, is not stringent enough to prevent the untimely clogging of arteries with plaque. A diet consisting of no more than 15-20% fat is more in line with the prevention of arterial plaque formation.

Let's examine some of these numbers and see how they relate. Let's say, for arguments sake, you consume 1600 calories a day. Fifteen to twenty percent of your 1600 calories would be between 240-320 calories per day. Well, that's great, but how much fat does that equate to? Fat is generally measured in grams. If you look on the back of food labels, you will see fat gram numbers per serving. A gram of fat yields approximately 9 calories. So, if you now look at your range of 240-320 calories to be made up of fat grams and divide the calories by 9, you will arrive at the number of fat grams per day you can consume while still remaining within your target of 15-20% of total calories. These calculations give you a fat gram range of approximately 27-36 grams a day, with a total calorie consumption of 1600 calories. Now these numbers will start to make some sense. The average American female consumes 2400 calories a day, and the average American male 3200 calories per day. To add insult to injury, the average American diet contains from 130-150 grams of fat per day.

If the average American is consuming approximately 140 grams of fat per day, how am I going to get down to 30-50 grams per day? The answer is by first being aware of how many fat grams the foods you eat contain, and then by making intelligent alternative choices. It is much easier today to find alternative fat substitutes than it was 10 years ago. We now have fat-free mayonnaise, fat-free salad dressing, fat-free yogurt, fat-free cookies, and even fat-free pastries. Most grocery stores also offer low-fat cheeses, salad dressings, margarines, snack foods and lunch meats. If you haven't counted fat grams before, you are not aware that the above-mentioned foods are extremely high in fat grams in their normal versions. Mayonnaise, for example, has 11 grams of fat per tablespoon, butter has 12, and oils about 14. So you can see that, if these three foods play a big part in your diet, it doesn't take long to get up to 150 grams of fat a day. These three foods may play a bigger part in your diet than you think, disguised in snack foods and desserts.

Snack foods play an important role in your daily fat consumption. For example, Keebler's *Pecan Sandies* contain 30 grams of fat in just 6 cookies. I know I can eat

6 *Pecan Sandies* in a heartbeat if I'm not careful. Many of the other snack cookies also have very high fat contents. A general rule you can apply is to look at the **high-calorie** snack foods as **high-fat** snack foods because, as you may remember, fat grams are high in calories.

I have listed above, as well as in *Tables 5.2 - 5.3*, some of the fat-free substitutes you can use as replacements for their normal versions. These substitutions alone will greatly reduce the number of fat grams per day you consume. Other substitutes which will help include low-fat margarines, such as *Diet Mazola* and *Promise Extra Light*, which contain 6 grams of fat per tablespoon instead of the 12 grams found in butter. For snacks, air popped popcorn or pretzels each have 1 gram or less of fat for a normal serving, instead of the 10-30 grams per serving found in many cookies and cakes. Instead of mayonnaise, which is high in fat, use mustard, taco sauce, horseradish, or ketchup, which have less than 1 gram of fat per tablespoon. You can see from the examples given that there are many choices for substitutes. All you really need to do is know the fat content of foods so that you can make intelligent alternative choices.

The following tables illustrate the fat content of some popular foods and condiments.

TABLE 5.2
FAT CONTENT OF CONDIMENTS

CONDIMENT	CALORIES	FAT (gm)
Mayonnaise	100	11
Salad Dressing	70	7
Reduced Cal Mayonnaise	50	5
Light Salad Dressing	45	4
Ketchup	16	<1
Pickle Relish	21	<1
Yellow Mustard	11	<1
Taco Sauce	4	<1

(Adapted from the University of California, Berkeley Wellness Letter 1987-1989)

TABLE 5.3
FAT CONTENT OF SNACK FOODS

DESCRIPTION	UNITS PER OZ.	KCAL	FAT (gm)
CRACKERS			
Rice Cakes (Quacker)	3	105	.02
Ry Krisp (Purina)	4	80	0.4
Melba Toast (Devonsheer)	10	112	0.5
Zwieback (Nabisco)	4	125	1.6
Wheat Thins (Interbake)	4	130	2.0
Saltines (Nabisco)	10	130	3.0
Graham (Nabisco)	4	120	3.0
Triscuit (Nabisco)	7	125	4.5
Ritz (Nabisco)	9	160	8.7
COOKIES			
Date Filled Oatmeal (Archway)	1	90	1
Fig Newton (Nabisco)	2	100	2
Molasses (Archway)	1	90	2
Ginger Snaps (Nabisco)	4	120	3
Cinnamon Graham (Keebler)	8	140	4
Amaranth (Health Valley)	2	140	6
Fruit Date (Health Valley)	2	140	6
Old Fashioned Oatmeal (Keebler)	2	160	6
Oreos (Nabisco)	3	140	6
Chips Ahoy (Nabisco)	3	140	7
Pecan Sandies (Keebler)	2	160	10
Almond Suprm (Peprdge Farm)	2	140	10
SNACK FOOD			
Popcorn (Plain)	4 cups	100	1
Pretzels	2 large	110	1
Tortilla or Corn Chips	1 oz.	155	8
Potato Chips	15 chips	160	10
Cheese Puffs or Twists	1 oz.	160	10

(Adapted from the University of California, Berkeley Wellness Letter 1987-1989)

Many studies have been conducted in a search to discover the contributing factors associated with the development of coronary heart disease. One such study that began in 1983 in Mainland China, demonstrates the relationship between the percentage of fat in the diet and heart disease. This study is currently being led by T. Colin Campbell, Ph.D., of the Division of Nutritional Sciences at Cornell University: To date, the study has involved more than 6,500 people from 65 different counties of Mainland China. One of the facts resulting from the study is that the people of China only consume 15% of their total calories from fat, as opposed to the 37-40% of total calories that we in the United States consume. This indicates that we are consuming double, and sometimes triple, the amount of total fat that the Chinese are. The study also indicates that 77% of the Chinese people's total calories come from complex carbohydrates, as opposed to 45% in the American diet.[11] With the high percentage of calories from complex carbohydrates, the Chinese consume about 35 grams of fiber per day, as opposed to the 10-12 grams for Americans. "When you eat a diet based on animal products -- as most Americans do -- you consume more fat and protein, and that can be a problem," says Brian Morgan, Ph.D., a Miami-based nutritionist.[12]

What are the consequences of these differences between our diets? One result of our dietary differences is a much lower blood cholesterol level for Chinese men. The mean cholesterol concentration for American men is 212 (milligrams per deciliter of blood) and, for rural Chinese men, it's between 135 and 140. Only 4 in every 100,000 adult males die of heart disease in China each year, as compared to 67 out of 100,000 in the United States. When it comes to women, the ratio of death from heart disease is 3 Chinese females to 19 American females.[13]

As you can see from the above-mentioned study,

the Chinese consume substantially more fiber than Americans do. Many studies have shown that fiber intake has an inverse relationship to heart disease. Certain types of fiber affect fat metabolism in a favorable way as it pertains to heart disease. Not all fibers have similar effects. For example, wheat bran, which is composed mostly of cellulose, has no cholesterol-lowering effect, whereas oat bran and the fiber of apples (pectin) do lower blood cholesterol. Fibers which form gels in water (pectin, guar and gum arabic) are the fibers which bind with bile salts and prevent them from producing cholesterol.[14]

So we can see that there is a strong correlation between the 37-40% of total calories from the fat which Americans consume and their relatively high incidence of coronary heart disease. On the other hand, we can see that the Chinese diet, which consists of about 15% fat out of their total calories, yields a relatively low incidence of heart disease.

So, now that we know that the *amount* of fat in our diet greatly affects our incidence of heart disease, what about the ***kind*** of fat we ingest? Does it really matter what kinds of fats we consume? It sure does! Not all fats are alike! Different kinds of fats have a different influence on our coronary arteries. Many studies have shown that excess saturated fat in the diet is the Number One villain in this crime scene. Recent research has been able to narrow the risk factors even more closely. Excess saturated fat raises total cholesterol, triglycerides and LDL to unhealthy levels. Even if we are consuming too much fat in proportion to total calories, we can improve our Blood Lipid Profile by substituting polyunsaturated and monounsaturated fats for much of our saturated fats. Polyunsaturated fats, in moderation, have been shown to lower total cholesterol levels in a beneficial way. Monounsaturated fats seem even more discriminatory. They not only lower total cholesterol but also lower LDL (the bad cholesterol) proportionately more than even polyunsaturated fats.

A study performed by Dr. Mensink and Dr. Katan highlights the specific actions of poly and monounsaturated fats. In their study, participants were first placed on a diet high in saturated fat for 17 days. In this diet, saturated fat accounted for 19.3% of the daily caloric intake; 11.5% was from monounsaturated fat; and 4.6% was from polyunsaturated fat. For the next 36 days, the group was placed on a mixed diet with the same total fat content. Half the group was randomly assigned to a diet containing a greater proportion of olive oil (monounsaturated fat) and the others were assigned to a diet enriched with sunflower oil (polyunsaturated fat).

The serum LDL cholesterol level decreased while the patients were on both low saturated fat diets. However, the serum LDL levels dropped 17.9% in the group on the monounsaturated fat diet, as opposed to 12.9% in the group on the polyunsaturated fat diet.[15] This study highlights the fact that, while replacing saturated fat in your diet with polyunsaturated fat is beneficial, you get the most benefit by switching to monounsaturated fat.

Exercise and Heart Disease

Exercise can play a major role in the prevention of heart disease. It can also influence a wide range of physical and emotional factors which dictate your heart disease risk level. One risk factor which contributes to heart attacks occurs when blood clots form inside blood vessels. These clots usually occur inside vessels which already have blockages from fatty deposits of cholesterol. When a clot forms inside an already clogged artery, the blood flow can be cut off, thus causing a heart attack or stroke.

Researchers at the University of Washington in Seattle have conducted studies which indicate that exercise can increase the production of a chemical produced by the blood vessels which actually dissolves clots.[16] Men between the ages of 25 and 74 participated in a 6-month study which included walking, jogging and bicycling. The program involved 30 to 45 minutes of exercise 4 to 5 days per week. At the end of the study period, the clot-dissolving chemical, tissue plasminogen activator, had increased by 29%. The increase of this anti-clogging chemical to such a degree represents a significant protective factor against heart attack or stroke.

High blood pressure is another risk factor of heart disease which can benefit from exercise. High blood pressure is caused by the constriction of the blood vessels, resulting in a higher than normal pressure pushing out on these vessels. Common sense tells you that if there is more pressure pushing out on these vessels, there is a greater chance of a blowout. Many factors influence the constriction of these blood vessels. One cause is a contraction of the tiny muscles on the inside walls of these vessels. Exercise can relax these muscles, thus relaxing the blood vessels and allowing them to expand and reduce the pressure. Exercise also reduces the level of certain hormones which constrict the blood vessels.[17] As blood vessel walls tend to become more rigid with age, exercise can also increase the flexibility of blood vessels, allowing them to expand and contract more readily.

What other factors play a significant role in the prevention of heart disease?

The Free Radical Theory

Well, let me start with a discussion about oxidation and the *Free Radical Theory*. These two phenomena play significant, everyday roles in many processes throughout your body. They affect every organ and system of your body in ways researchers are only beginning to understand.

Life as we know it is mostly dependent on the availability of oxygen. Life would not exist for more than a few minutes if oxygen suddenly disappeared. In recent years, we have been indoctrinated with the knowledge that aerobic (the use of oxygen) exercise is extremely beneficial in maintaining overall fitness, and cardiac fitness in particular. While this is true enough, what is also true is that oxygen causes a degrading effect on all organs of the body. But if it's true that we need oxygen in order to live, how can it be bad for us? Well, let me answer that with a question. What happens to a piece of iron left outside in the air? What about rubber or wood? All of these things "oxidize." Oxidation is a chemical process catalyzed by oxygen wherein one substance degrades into another. The burning of gasoline or wood is an oxidation reaction.

So, in similar fashion, oxygen is harmful to our bodily systems by participating in the degrading process of our tissues and organs. Oxidation damage creates uncontrolled molecular particles called *free radicals* which travel randomly inside the body. Researchers theorize that these so-called free radicals are at least partly responsible for the way our skin becomes leathery and also for the development of cataracts as we age. In fact, the damage these free radicals do to our tissues and organs is believed to play a heavy role in the aging process. What we may believe to be normal aging of all humans is, in fact, premature destruction of our tissues and organs due to the oxidative damage of free radicals. It is the damage done at the cellular level which is of most concern. Free radicals react with fats in cell membranes and destroy them through peroxidation, which is a process similar to that which turns butter rancid.[18]

Recently, scientists have put forth a new theory on how cholesterol can penetrate and clog arterial walls. In the early 1980s, scientists began to investigate the relationship between free radicals and LDL cholesterol (the bad kind). For years, scientists had suspected that LDL itself wasn't causing the damage in heart disease. The damage resulted from something happening to LDL in the bloodstream. And that "something," they theorized, might be free radicals damaging LDL. In the bloodstream, only oxidized (not normal) LDL is taken up by macrophages (cells which eat other cells), which convert it to material that can be deposited in the arteries. So the presence of oxidized LDL may promote the accumulation of arteriosclerotic plaque -- the beginning phase of heart disease.[19]

Supplementation

Your body has an elaborate system for handling oxidation reactions, if only you give it the raw materials to engage the battle. The raw materials needed are called "antioxidants." We should get them mainly through our diets. It may be prudent to supplement our diets with some of the most potent antioxidants. Vitamins C and E, along with beta carotene and selenium, are the most talked about antioxidants by researchers. A word of caution: supplements are by no means a ***replacement*** for obtaining antioxidants through a proper diet. A diet consisting mostly of fruits, vegetables, nuts and seeds, with animal products as side dishes, will provide you with ample antioxidant protection.

In a study reported in *Atherosclerosis*, a respected periodical on heart disease, scientists performed a test tube study showing the correlation between antioxidants in the blood and oxidation damage to human cholesterol. The study demonstrated Vitamins C and E's ability to stop oxidation and, consequently, free radical development in test tube samples of human blood cholesterol.[20] It is believed that cholesterol must be oxidized before it begins to invade the arterial walls. If this theory holds true, then ensuring that your diet provides abundant supplies of antioxidants may enable you to effectively block the formation of arterial plaques.

There are many factors that make up our complex antioxidant system. Vitamins A, E, and C, along with the minerals, zinc and selenium, supported by the activity of numerous enzymes, make up the bulk of what we know today about this system. If we add fruits and vegetables which are highest in known antioxidant properties, we can be assured of getting some measure of protection from the damage caused by oxidation. Citrus fruits, along with strawberries and cantaloupe, contain large amounts of Vitamin C. The dark yellow and orange fruits and vegetables, as well as dark green leafy vegetables, contain ample supplies of beta carotene. Some examples of beta carotene rich foods are apricots, pumpkin, carrots, squash, spinach and broccoli. Vegetables of all colors supply Vitamin E.[21]

In many animal studies, supplementation with antioxidants has yielded beneficial results. Supplementation also seems to has positive effects on humans. Based on the results of such studies, it appears prudent to supplement one's diet with additional antioxidants. The ones researchers know the most about are Vitamins A, C, and E, as well as selenium. [A note of caution: Vitamin A in its standard form can be toxic in large doses. It is better to use beta-carotene, which has not been shown to be toxic in large doses.]

Dr. Lynos Pauling, the undeniably brilliant scientist and author who has won two Nobel Prizes for his contributions to science, has contended for years that heart disease is predominantly a Vitamin C deficiency disease. He claims that Vitamin C plays several roles in our protection against heart disease.* First of all, Vitamin C is a powerful antioxidant. Antioxidants, as I said earlier, help prevent the formation of free radicals which are believed to damage the arterial walls and oxidize fats (hence, clogging the arteries). Pauling also believes that Vitamin C is a big healer of all kinds of tissues, including capillaries. So, if we have little scars or injuries on the insides of our arteries, Vitamin C will heal these damaged arteries. Recent tests have also indicated that Vitamin C will elevate your good cholesterol (HDL) level.

In Dr. Pauling's most recent research study, he claims to have found that the real culprit in heart disease is not LDL, but is instead a lipoprotein called LPA (Lipoprotein A). These small particles of LPA resemble LDL cholesterol, but are the real culprits which stick to the arterial walls and cause damage. LPA and Vitamin C are both attracted to injuries in the arteries in the same way. So, if your concentration of Vitamin C is high enough, it will fill in and heal the cracked and damaged portions of the arteries before the LPA can get in there and cause a blockage. Dr. Pauling believes that if you take enough Vitamin C, through both diet and supplementation, you can eliminate this LPA damage.

The reason I sound a little ambivalent about supplementation is because supplements should be **extra** nutritional insurance, not an excuse for poor eating habits. Supplements are not a replacement for altering one's diet to include an ample supply of antioxidants.

---

*Unfortunately, the medical profession has not yet recognized Dr. Pauling's claims regarding Vitamin C. Mayo Clinic did a study some years ago on the effects of Vitamin C on cancer. They concluded from this "study" that there was no evidence that Vitamin C helped terminally ill cancer patients. In response, Dr. Pauling said, "Well, you can't radiate them up, shoot them up with poisons, and then think that Vitamin C is going to do any good after you've destroyed their immune system with all that." Dr. Pauling, however, has had many positive results with Vitamin C treatment for cancer patients, including significant extensions of their lives after treatment.

Supplementation is not an exact science. Who could possibly believe that a vitamin supplement manufactured by man could contain all the intricate molecular particles and relationships that nature has contrived in the formulation of its vitamins in whole foods? This fact is highlighted by the continuous discovery of additional nutrient co-factors found in foods by researchers. So, if you want to add some supplementation of antioxidants to your diet as an insurance policy, that's fine. But don't expect the supplements to create miracles while you continue poor eating habits. In your search for supplements, keep in mind that liquid or powder supplements are better than those found in tablet form since liquids and powders are more easily and quickly absorbed into the bloodstream. Tablets and capsules are often eliminated from the body whole, not absorbed at all.

***Table 5.4* highlights my recommended daily supplementation schedule.**

TABLE 5.4
DAILY SUPPLEMENT GUIDE

SUPPLEMENT	DAILY SUPPLEMENTATION AMOUNT
Beta-Carotene	25,000 I. U.
Vitamin C	1,000 - 3,000 Mg. (Ascorbate Form) *
Vitamin E	200 - 400 I.U.
Selenium	100 - 150 Mcg. *
Zinc	15 - 30 Mg.
Copper	1 - 2 Mg. *

*Ascorbate forms of Vitamin C are combined with a mineral transporter, such as calcium, to facilitate absorption.
*Selenium can be toxic above 200 mcg. per day
*Zinc supplementation should be accompanied with copper because zinc competes with copper for absorption.

These doses are fairly conservative and appear to be without any noticeable side effects. Higher doses have been recommended by some authoritative proponents of antioxidants. They could very well be right. If you feel you would like higher levels of antioxidants in your blood, try to increase your dietary sources. There are many other antioxidants, both in your diet and in supplemental form. Researchers are at this time unraveling the mystery surrounding many of these. I am sure we will be hearing more about many of them in the near future.

What Can We Do to Reverse Heart Disease?

Much has been discussed about preventing heart disease, but what about reversing its effects once we have it? Is it possible? Recent studies appear to indicate just that.

One of the most widely-cited evidences showing reversal of atherosclerosis in humans is Dr. Blankenhorn's 1987 study, which showed that, for every one percent reduction in blood cholesterol, heart attack risk decreases by two percent. For example, if your blood cholesterol level is 200 mg/dl, and you reduce it to 198 mg/dl (a 1% reduction) you will reduce your risk of having a heart attack by 2%. More importantly, the study demonstrated that if serum cholesterol declines enough, plaques occluding the arteries can actually reduce in size.[22]

In Dr. Blankenhorn's 1987 study, he divided his patients into two groups. One group received very high doses of cholesterol-lowering drugs, and the second group did not receive the drugs. Both groups followed the American Heart Association's recommendation of no more than 30% total dietary fat. The patients on the cholesterol-lowering drugs showed a decrease of blood cholesterol to below the 180 mark. But only 16% of the patients using cholesterol-lowering drugs showed any measurable **reversal** of their coronary artery blockage.[23] This suggests that lowering your blood cholesterol alone is not significant enough to cause reversal of existing arterial blockages.

In contrast to Dr. Blankenhorn's study, Dr. Dean Ornish, from the University of California at San Francisco, has conducted a study in which 82% of the patients who followed his program for a year showed shrinkage of their coronary artery blockages. Dr. Dean Ornish's program involves reducing dietary fat to 10% of total calories on a vegetarian diet. He also advocates no smoking or drinking of caffeinated beverages. In his program, he also stresses the need for 30 minutes of exercise at least six times a week, plus stress-reduction exercises. People who faithfully follow his program have shown remarkable progress in not only halting arterial blockages but in actually reversing it.

Exercise. Animal studies indicate that exercise can not only help prevent clogged arteries, as discussed previously, but can actually help reverse them. At the very least, exercise can stimulate the growth of new collateral blood vessels. These blood vessels branch out from the original blood vessel as a result of extra demand for blood flow caused by exercise. If you exercise regularly, the muscles and tissues used during this activity demand a greater blood flow. This additional blood flow is needed to deliver fuel to the muscles and to remove waste products from them. The heart is the beneficiary of this more efficient blood delivery system. With additional collateral blood vessels available, there is less chance of a fatal heart attack from a clogged artery.

CANCER

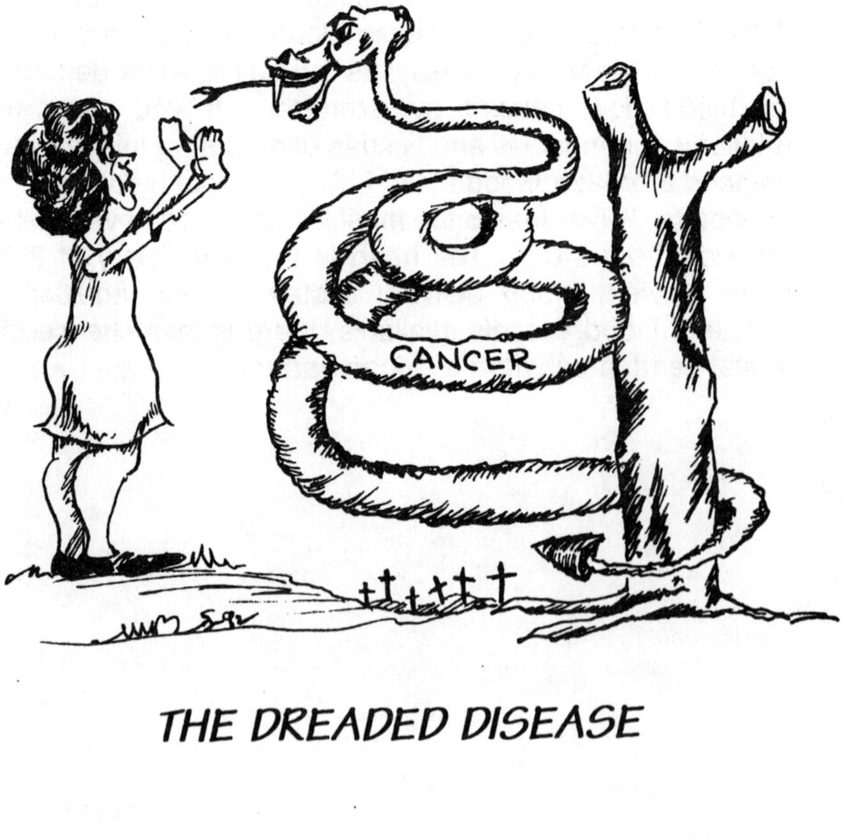

THE DREADED DISEASE

Chapter 6

CANCER

THE word "cancer" itself instills fear in every person's mind. It is the one disease universally dreaded by all societies. In society today, cancer instills the same fear as did the bubonic plague of the Middle Ages, or as leprosy did in Biblical times. It is estimated that about 73 million people living today will eventually develop cancer. Three out of four families will be affected.[1] Cancer is the Number Two killer in our society today, surpassed only by heart disease.

The main reason for the tremendous fear associated with cancer is due to lack of knowledge. Most people simply don't understand what cancer really is. They don't know that 80 to 90 percent of cancers are due to environmental factors mostly in their control. Of course there are certain environmental factors beyond our control, such as being close to a nuclear reactor when it melts down, as in the Chernobyl incident. But, for the most part, we can control, or at least channel, most environmental factors if we have knowledge of their danger. Diet is one of the most important contributing environmental factors to the development of cancer in our society today. The amount of fat you eat greatly determines your cancer risk for many of the high mortality cancers. World population studies support these facts. The countries that have the highest consumption of daily fat have the highest incidences of breast and colon cancer. On the contrary, the countries that have the lowest consumption of daily fat have the lowest incidences of these two cancers. Although there are other environmental factors which affect your chances of developing cancer, if you control your dietary fat intake and eliminate cigarette smoking, you will greatly reduce your chances of developing the high mortality cancers.

If lack of knowledge is contributing to our fear of this dreaded affliction, then it is time to define this disease. I will present an overview of what the disease is and how it is believed to develop.

What Is Cancer?

Cancer is a common term used to describe a subgroup of a class of diseases formally called "neoplasms." Cancer refers to the most aggressive, and sometimes fatal, sub-group of neoplasms. Some neoplasms develop into non-malignant cysts or tumors. Therefore, all neoplasms are not cancerous. A neoplasm is classified as either benign or malignant. A benign neoplasm is encapsulated, its malignant counterpart is not. Malignant neoplasms tend to grow more rapidly and invade nearby healthy tissue. Benign tumors appear similar to the host tissue from which it originated. Malignant tumors or neoplasms appear totally different from the host tissue it originated from. The most distinct characteristic that distinguishes the two types of neoplasms is the tendency of malignant neoplasms to spread or metastasize at sites other than where they originated from.

Cancer cells act independently from the surrounding tissue or organs. Cancer cells do not obey the natural laws of growth and metabolism. Most cells of the body work in unison with other cells in the form of a distinct tissue or organ for the benefit of the body as a whole. Cancerous cells act completely independent from the host organ or tissue creating a neoplasm with uncontrolled growth resulting in harm to the body as a whole.

Initiation and Promotion

Let's talk about how malignant neoplasms or cancers develop. This is the area where we can exert considerable influence into preventing the onset of cancer in ourselves. Contrary to the popular belief that cancer is in our genes, and we have no control over getting it, cancer is, for the most part, controllable and preventable. Cancer is generally believed to develop in a two-step process. The first stage of cancer development occurs when some type of radiation or chemical carcinogen intrudes into a cell. This first stage is called the *Initiation Stage*. This stage is believed to be irreversible. This Initiation Stage in itself does not cause the growth of a cancerous neoplasm.

Cancer growth requires a second stage in order to start the growth of a malignant neoplasm. This second stage is called the *Promotion Stage*. Promotion requires the introduction of a second agent known as the promoting agent. Unlike the Initiation Stage of cancer, promotion is controllable and reversible. The cells must be exposed to the promoting agent or agents many times before cancer begins to develop. Furthermore, if the cells are exposed to the promoting agents over long intervals instead of short intervals, cancerous neoplasms do not develop. If the promoting agents invade the cells at frequent intervals, they may alter the DNA structure of the cell. The DNA contains the genetic blueprint for the reproduction of cells from one generation to another. If the promoting agent alters this blueprint substantially, a mutant cell will be produced during cell division.

If you followed the Initiation and Promotion Stages just outlined, you can see that we have considerable control over the Promotion Stage of the development of cancer. Remember, cancer will not begin to develop until the second agent bombards the cells, not once, but many times. Even if the second agent is placed in contact with the cells, it will not cause the development of the cancerous tumor if the frequency of exposure is spread out far enough.

Promoting Agents

Dietary fat, excessive animal protein, alcoholic beverages, cigarette smoke, and several food additives are promoting agents in everyone's control. There have been many studies conducted by notable scientists whose works can substantiate these allegations.

One such study, conducted by Paolo Toniolo, an epidemiologist at New York University Medical Center, in conjunction with the International Agency for Research on Cancer in Lyon, France, has shown a definite link between diet and cancer, especially breast cancer. The conclusion drawn from the evidence displayed in the study is that saturated fats and animal proteins are the most potent risk factors to the development of breast cancer.

The research group compared the diets of 250 breast cancer patients against those of 499 healthy women of about the same age, based on questionnaires regarding foods and portions eaten. The questionnaires have revealed that the breast cancer patients typically consume higher percentages of fat and protein than the healthy women. To be more specific, the higher percentages were made up entirely of a higher consumption of meat and dairy products, specifically more milk, high-fat cheese, and butter.[2]

The research group goes on to further clarify its findings by concluding that breast cancer risk was three times greater than normal for the women who consumed about half their calories as fat, 13 to 23 percent of their calories as saturated fat, and 8 to 20 percent of their calories as animal protein. The women in the group who limited their saturated fat intake to less than 10 percent of calories or animal protein to less than 6 percent of calories, had half the breast cancer risk typical for this region.[3]

Cancer risk increases relatively with increases in fat consumption. If you are on a relatively low-fat diet, if you increase your fat consumption, your cancer risk will increase proportionately.

A new Chinese study illustrates the fact that the risk of breast cancer rises with an increase in fat consumption. Study participants averaged 22.7 percent of their calories from fat, whereas Americans average 38 - 40 %.

Researchers from Shanghai Medical University and Canada's National Cancer Institute in Toronto interviewed 186 women with breast cancer, 186 healthy women living in the same urban Shanghai neighborhoods, and 186 women hospitalized nearby with other malignancies associated with different risk factors. The 20 percent who consumed the most calories (a daily average of 3,142) and fat (34 percent of calories), had nearly double the breast cancer risk than the 20 percent who consumed the fewest calories (1,733) and least fat (13.8 percent).[4] While the Shanghai women consumed nearly 70 percent of their fat calories in the form of monounsaturates, the North Americans consumed about 44 percent from monounsaturated fats and another 44 percent from saturated fats. Together with the Western findings, the new Chinese data suggest that for breast cancer risk, the **quantity** of fat consumed matters more than the **type** of fat selected.[5]

Another factor under your control which appears to have a high incidence of cancer associated with it, is cooked sugar, or protein cooked in fat. Cooking food is often deleterious to your health. I am sorry to tell you that your holiday barbecue is probably loaded with fat that is lining the insides of your arteries with plaque, thus contributing to your demise through heart disease. To add insult to injury, this same grilled steak, or even chicken, is probably acting as a promoting agent in the formation of cancerous cells. We have now learned that cooked meat is a cancer promoter on two counts: its fat content, and its cooked protein factor.

A study conducted by W. Robert Bruce investigated the relationship between cooking and colon cancer. He and his colleagues discovered that cooking transforms benign ingredients into compounds that promote the growth of colon tumors that can turn into malignancies. Working at the Ontario Cancer Institute in Toronto, the researchers chemically induced small tumors in the colons of 152 mice and 83 rats. Then they fed the animals diets differing only in whether the sugar, protein, or fat had been cooked (to 324 F). After 100 days, animals whose diets contained either cooked sugar or protein cooked in fat showed three to five times as many large, precancerous tumors as any in the other groups. The findings, Bruce says, suggest that by-products of the cooked sucrose and casein can promote colon cancer development. Fat, by itself, also poses a risk, he notes, pointing to previous work in which his group found that animals on diets with 20 percent fat showed a 50 percent increase in tumor development, compared with animals receiving 5 percent fat. However, he says, the fat risk was clearly much smaller than that associated with cooked casein or sucrose. The Toronto team is now trying to identify the cancer-promoting by-products in the cooked sugar and protein.[6]

The Secret is to Prevent

So, what's the first step toward cancer prevention? First of all, you must analyze your diet so that you know where you stand with respect to your dietary fat and protein consumption. After you've made a thorough examination of your diet, you can then begin to make the necessary alterations.

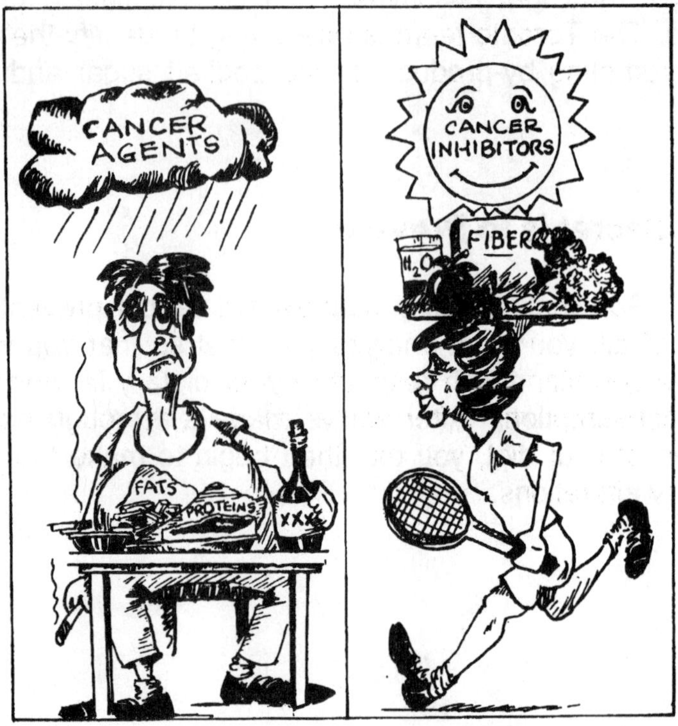

Now let's discuss some beneficial components you can add to your diet which will not only prevent the formation of cancer, but may be able to short-circuit cancer if it is in its beginning stages. There are many new theories arising from the research front and many new anti-cancer inhibitors being touted as the cure-all. I will try to help you make sense of a few of the more promising ones.

These are exciting times for the researchers, but they may also be confusing times for the layperson what with enough theories floating around to confuse even the most astute of students. Out of all this research, a common consensus is beginning to emerge. Let's look at some of the more promising conclusions.

Antioxidants and Cancer

Do you remember our discussions of heart disease and the Free Radical Theory? Well, the Free Radical Theory also applies to cancer formation. Some of the initiators and promoters of cancer are created by the oxidation of compounds in the bloodstream by free radicals. These free radicals are highly reactive with fats in the body. Cell membranes contain a high proportion of fat which reacts with these free radicals, initiating the process of cancer formation. The nervous system and the brain also contain a rich supply of lipids subject to free radical destruction.

If damage is done to cells around the body by oxidation, then antioxidants are at least part of the key to preventing some of this damage. In fact, numerous studies performed by scientists around the world strongly lead to this conclusion. Study after study has linked beta-carotene, Vitamins C, E and the trace mineral selenium with lower incidence of cancer. There are many other organic compounds found in foods which are emerging from recent research as potent cancer inhibitors that will be made public in the near future. In the meantime, eat plenty of fruits and vegetables of all colors, and you will be receiving the benefits of this new research before the general public is made aware.

The theory that antioxidants can play a beneficial role in health is not a new theory. This theory has been circulating around for more than thirty years. What is new about it is that organizations like the National Cancer Institute and the World Health Organization are becoming strong believers in it. In 1990, the World Health Organization held a conference specifically on antioxidants. This conference was attended by 36 of the world's leading research scientists in this field. They discussed the role of the antioxidants in preventing degenerative diseases.

They stated that antioxidants exerted a protective influence on cells by blocking cell damage from the effects of free radical oxidative reactions that take place during metabolism. The scientists highlighted the fact that different antioxidants played individual roles in their protection of oxidative damage. For example, Vitamin E, a fat-soluble vitamin, acts as a free radical scavenger and protects the fats in cell membranes. Vitamin C, which is water-soluble, serves a similar function in cellular fluids.[7] Numerous scientists from around the world have reported the results of studies which confirm the relationship between cancer prevention and elevated blood levels of the antioxidants.

One study, reviewed by George W. Comstock, Ph.D., of Johns Hopkins University in Baltimore, Maryland, reviewed data from a previous study in 1974, where 26,000 people donated blood samples to a blood bank. These blood samples were analyzed for nutrients, hormones, antibodies and other factors. The people who volunteered the blood were watched for years to track their disease incidence. When enough cancers were reported in the donors, their blood was cross-matched for various components such as antioxidants to see if there were any correlations. The data showed a strong inverse association between the amount of beta-carotene in the blood and the risk of lung cancer, as well as an association between low levels of Vitamin E and lung cancer.[8] Other excerpts from prominent scientists attending the World Health Conference are as follows:

"In both prospective and retrospective epidemiologic studies, low dietary intake of fruits and vegetables (carotenoids) is associated with an increased risk of lung cancer", according to Regina G. Ziegler, Ph.D., M.P.H. of the National Cancer Institute, Bethesda, Maryland.[9] "Diet does not necessarily eliminate the risk of lung cancer attributable to smoking," she said, "but the levels of carotenoid intake characteristic of about 30 percent of a typical community may be sufficient for a noticeable reduction -- 25 to 55 percent -- in lung cancer risk".[10]

"There is evidence of a possible protective role for Vitamin E in various cancers which affect women," said Paul Knekt, Ph.D., of the Social Insurance Institution, Helsinki, Finland, at the conference. Analysis of stored blood samples from cancer patients and controls revealed that women with the lowest levels of Vitamin E in their blood had 1.6 times the risk of cancer as those with higher levels. Women with low levels of Vitamin E and selenium, (the mineral that is also an antioxidant) had 10 times the breast cancer risk.[11]

Studies have also shown the effects of the antioxidants Vitamins A, C and E on the development of polyps of the colon. The antioxidants significantly reduced the rate of recurrence of removed polyps in high risk individuals. These polyps, when they recur, may eventually become cancerous. Anything that can reduce their recurrence also reduces the risk of possible cancer.

So what can you do with this information? Just as you will need to analyze your diet for fat and protein content, you must also analyze your diet for antioxidant containing foods. Many of the orange and yellow fruits and vegetables are good sources of the antioxidants. (See *Table 6.1*). But all fruits and vegetables contain factors that act, if not as antioxidants, as other types of cancer inhibitors.

TABLE 6.1
ANTIOXIDANT SOURCES

FOOD ITEM	QUANTITY	VITAMIN A (RE) *	VITAMIN C (mg)
Most Foods Contain 2 Antioxidants			
Sweet Potato,Peeled	1 Medium	2480	28
Cantaloupe	1/2 Large	865	115
Broccoli	1 Cup	222	97
Carrot, Whole	1 Whole	2025	10
Papaya, Raw	1/2 Large	408	112
Brussel Sprouts	1 Cup	114	97
Strawberries/sliced	1 Cup	7	120
Mango, Fresh	1 Medium	806	57
Orange	1 Medium	27	70
Parsley, Chopped	1 Cup	312	54
Collards, Cooked	1 Cup	1017	45
Blackberries	1 Cup	24	30
Green Pepper	1 Pod	39	95
Watermelon	2" by 10"	350	94
Cauliflower	1 Cup	T	69
Asparagus, Cooked	1 Cup	150	

Adapted from: Understanding Normal & clinical Nutrition, Whitney, Cataldo, Rolfes, 1987
* (RE) Stands for the term Retinol Equivalent. 1 RE = approximately 5 - I.U.

Table 6.1 presents some dietary sources of the antioxidants, beta carotene and Vitamin C. It is important to incorporate many of these food sources into your daily diet. Along with these two antioxidants, you should incorporate 3 to 4 ounces of raw fresh seeds and nuts in your diet per week. The seeds and nuts, along with vegetable oils, are good sources of the antioxidant Vitamin E. You should be careful, however, with the quantity of these food items you consume on a daily basis, since the nuts, seeds, and oils also contain a generous portion of fat.

Are you beginning to see a pattern here? Earlier, I discussed the hypothesis put forward by many scientists that LDLs, (Low Density Lipoproteins), the bad cholesterol, begin to cause damage to artery walls and create plaques that eventually clog the arteries only after oxidative damage from free radicals occurs. To put it in simpler terms, clogging of arteries only occurs after damage from free radicals to the cholesterol and artery walls. On the seemingly other end of the disease spectrum, you have cancer being greatly inhibited by prevention of oxidative damage from the same free radicals. There's the link: oxidative damage through the action of free radical molecules causing or greatly influencing heart disease and cancer. To add icing to the cake, the fats circulating in the blood (LDLs) and the fats in cell membranes are the most susceptible to free radical damage.

In summary, oxidative damage, through the derangement of free radical molecules, greatly influences the formation of heart disease and cancer. The greater percentage of fat in the diet, the greater the risk of free radical damage to fats circulating in the blood and in the cell walls. With this knowledge, we can understand the need to limit dietary fat and increase dietary intake of antioxidant-containing foods.

Fiber and Cancer

Your dietary intake of fiber is another factor in your cancer risk. Studies have shown that a diet high in fiber, specifically insoluble fiber, can give us some protection from colon and rectal cancers. These types of cancer are the second leading cause of cancer deaths in the United States.[12] It is theorized that diets high in insoluble fiber (that which is found in wheat bran and whole grains) offer some protection from colon and rectal cancers by increasing the transit speed of food through the intestines. This increased flow of food out of the bowel decreases the time in which possible carcinogens come in contact with the bowel wall, thus decreasing the likelihood of cancerous mutations of the bowel wall cells. Other theories of how fiber assists in the prevention of bowel cancer involve the belief that fiber may dilute, bind, or inactivate cancer causing agents, thus reducing the risk of developing cancerous mutations of the cells lining the bowel.[13] The diluting or binding effect of some fibers is a characteristic of another type of fiber called soluble fiber. The soluble fibers are the gums and pectins found in fruits, vegetables, seeds, legumes, oats, and barley. These gums and pectins form gels when mixed with water.[14] It is theorized that these gels can bind with bile acids and lipids, thus carrying them out of the body. You may recall that oxidative damage through the actions of free radicals is a significant risk factor in the development of cancerous cell mutations. If the gels of the soluble fibers can reduce the amount of circulating fat molecules, then the fibers can contribute to a reduced bowel cancer risk.

The question is how much fiber should we eat daily? Just analyze the diets of people from countries around the world where cancer is lowest. In some regions of China, the people consume over 70 grams of fiber per day. Americans consume about 12 grams of fiber on a daily basis. Americans need to greatly increase their daily fiber intake to achieve the relatively low cancer rates of the Chinese. *Table 6.2* gives you some high fiber choices from foods which are desirable, not only for their fiber content, but also for the many other beneficial nutrients (such as antioxidants) they contain.

TABLE 6.2
HIGH FIBER FOODS

FOOD ITEM	QUANTITY	FIBER (gm)	CALORIES
Foods Listed by Highest Fiber Per Serving			
Figs, Dried	10 Each	24	480
Kidney Beans	1 Cup	20	230
Pinto Beans	1 Cup	19	265
Prunes	10 Each	13.5	200
Black Beans	1 Cup	15	190
Great Northern Beans	1 Cup	12.5	210
All Bran Cereal	1/2 Cup	12	105
Blackberries	1 Cup	10	80
Black Eyed Peas	1 Cup	10	190
Lentils	1 Cup	10	215
Apples, Dried	10 Each	9	150
Raspberries	1 Cup	9	60
Oatmeal	1 Cup	9	145
Garbanzo Beans	1 Cup	8.5	270
Dates	10 Each	7	230
Broccoli, Cooked	1 Cup	6.5	45
Apple, Whole	1 Each	4-6	80-120
Pears	1 Each	5	98
Raisins	1/2 Cup	5	215
Strawberries/Sliced	1 Cup	5	68
Watermelon	2" by 4	5	30
Brussel Sprouts	1 Cup	5	65
Baked Potato/skin	1 Each	4.5	220
Sweet Potato, Peeled	1 Each	4	120
Parsley, Chopped	1 Cup	4	20
Collards	1 Cup	4	60
Apricot Halves	10 Each	3.5	80
Mango, Whole	1 Medium	3	135
Orange, Whole	1 Medium	3	60
Pineapple, Chunks	1 Cup	3	76
Asparagus, Cooked	1 Cup	3	44

Exercise and Cancer

Everywhere we turn, exercise seems to have its finger in every pie. Exercise has been shown to benefit just about every system of the body, from the circulatory system to the muscular and the nervous systems. Research seems to highlight newly discovered links with exercise almost every week and keeps pinning new medals on the benefits of a regular exercise program. Regular exercise has been claimed to influence cardiac fitness, lower blood pressure, keep muscles and bones strong, and lower your stress levels. New research is indicating that regular exercise has a hand in cancer prevention.

One study, involving several thousand Japanese men, concluded that the men who were physically active had only half to three quarters the risk of developing colon cancer than that of sedentary men. The risk of developing colon cancer decreased as the resting heart rate of the men decreased.[15] In case you were unaware, regular aerobic exercise has the effect of lowering your resting heart rate. The lowering of your resting heart rate is one way exercise benefits your heart muscle in general. When your resting heart rate is 60 beats per minute instead of 80, your heart is working more efficiently, with more time to rest between beats.

Another study pointing to lowered cancer risk was conducted at Harvard and involved 5,000 former women athletes. The women who were athletes in their college years had lower incidences of breast, colon, thyroid, bladder and lung cancers than the average population, adjusted for age and sex.[16] Rose Frisch, Ph.D., Associate Professor of Population Sciences at the Harvard Center for Population Studies, theorizes that athletes have more active immune systems than non-athletes. Laboratory studies have indicated that exercise increases the action of "T" cells (cells in the immune system which seek and destroy foreign matter such as tumor cells), thus heightening the immune response.[17]

So it appears that if you increase your cardiovascular fitness with an exercise program which eventually lowers your resting heart rate, you will get the added bonus of lowered cancer risk, plus an increased immune function with far-reaching consequences.

New On the Horizon: Designer Foods

There is an explosion of research being conducted on the links between diet and disease. Scientists all around the world, almost simultaneously, are discovering strong links between the two. The National Cancer Institute has begun extensive studies on compounds found in certain plant foods. Researchers, like Herbert Pierson, at the National Cancer Institute, have discovered that many populations which consume substantial quantities of green, leafy vegetables, fruits, and grains, appear to have considerable protection from cancer. The scientists decided to attempt to isolate the plant compounds in the green, leafy vegetables, fruits, and grains that are responsible for this cancer protection. They have isolated a group of compounds they call *phytochemicals.*

Numerous animal studies have been conducted in which strong chemical carcinogens were administered to the test animals, along with many of the phytochemicals. These plant compounds exhibited strong anti-cancer protection to the animals. The research concluded that these phytochemicals affect, in a favorable way, human biochemical pathways.[18] The phytochemicals appear to trigger the activation of enzymes that help retard the formation of cancerous tumors. Scientists have been able to isolate and identify many of these plant compounds. The carotenoids are a good example of these phytochemicals. There are over 500 known carotenoids, of which beta carotene is the most recognizable. Also identified are the terpenoids, flavonoids, coumarins, indoles, and isothiocyanates.[19]

Examples of some foods which contain phytochemicals include the cruciferous vegetables (broccoli, cauliflower and brussels sprouts) that contain indoles. Indoles are believed to activate enzymes that break down carcinogens. Indoles also switch on enzymes that dismantle the female hormone, estrogen. The dismantling of estrogen may help protect against breast cancer.[20] Another example is flavonoids found in citrus fruits. Flavonoids are classified among the antioxidants which protects cells from free radicals.

All these phytochemicals are found in the foods we eat. The problem is that the quantities of these plant compounds in the foods we eat is so variable that you are never sure what quantity of phytochemical you are receiving at any given meal. A group of scientists decided to create foods with known quantities of the plant compounds and called them "designer foods."

The scientists at the National Cancer Institute are working diligently on this project. They hope within the next few years to be able to provide us with high potency, flavorful "designer foods" which offer substantial protection from cancer.

Chapter 7

OSTEOPOROSIS

OSTEOPOROSIS, the silent killer, is often overlooked by most people as a serious health threat. Most people also mistakenly believe that this disease affects only women. Men, women and children of all ages can be affected by this disease. The degree to which this disease is prevalent is alarming. Osteoporosis is not caused by any one factor but by a wide range of influences and living patterns.

Osteoporosis is characterized by a demineralization of the bones over a period of time. This loss of minerals in the bone structure results in hollow, weakened areas of the bone which are potential fracture sites. This disease won't kill you directly, but it will immobilize you so that other secondary diseases such as pneumonia can do their work.

How Serious a Threat is Osteoporosis?

Osteoporosis affects an incredible 15 to 20 million women who have gone through menopause. That's one-third of all postmenopausal females in the United States.[1] According the the *New England Journal of Medicine*, osteoporosis is responsible for at least 1.2 million bone fractures in the United States each year, with the vertebrae, the hip, and the forearm near the wrist being the most common sites.[2] By the time they reach old age, one-third of all women and one-sixth of all men will have had a hip fracture. Even more disturbing is the fact that these hip fractures are fatal 12 to 20 percent of the time.[3]

Don't underestimate the severity of this disease.

Lola's Story

Let me tell you a story about a woman named Lola. Most of us don't get the privilege of knowing our great grandparents. Well, I was one of those lucky few. You see, Lola was my great grandmother.

Lola lived in the Philippines in a rural setting. The diet and lifestyle of that country is vastly different from that of industrialized countries such as America. Lola's diet consisted of a lot of complex carbohydrates, such as rice and potatoes. Meat was usually an extra or sidedish, if at all. Her lifestyle, especially when she was young, was one of outdoor physical activity, centered around providing the necessities of life.

Up until the age of 98, Lola was a strong, healthy, vigorous women, free of any health problems. When she was 98, she broke her hip. She was confined to her bed for a month when she developed pneumonia and died shortly thereinafter. Well, you might say, at least she lived a long, fruitful life. True enough. But the shame of it is that she had absolutely no apparent health problems before her hip fracture. There is every reason to believe that, without the hip fracture, she may have lived another five to ten years.

The story of Lola is not one of tragedy. After all, she did live until her 99th birthday. The events which led to Lola's eventual death, however, are not uncommon. But the difference between Lola and other hip fracture victims is age. Most hip fracture victims are in their sixties or seventies, not their nineties like Lola was. It is tragic indeed for an otherwise healthy person to die of the complications of a hip fracture.

Osteoporosis does kill. Although it may not do so directly, it's deadly just the same. But it doesn't have to be this way. We can successfully alter our diets and living patterns to greatly reduce the influence of this killer disease. We must do something early in life to build the kind of frame that will withstand the tests of time. Let's now look at some of the basics.

What Are Bones Anyway?

Most of us think of bones as hard, rock-like substances in the body which are, once formed, inert matter subject to little change. Bones are, in fact, dynamic, living, changing tissue, much like the other tissues in the body.

Bone tissue is constantly being broken down and built up by special bone cells called osteoclasts and osteoblasts. The breaking down activity of the osteoclasts is triggered by hormones of the parathyroid and thyroid glands, along with prostaglandin from the bone cells themselves. If the thyroid or parathyroid become too active, the breakdown of bone may exceed the buildup process and cause a net loss of bone. Many factors can influence the excess secretion of hormone from these glands which would adversely affect proper bone formation. The incredibly sophisticated and intricate body perceives this danger and produces additional hormones in the thyroid gland to counteract the effects of too large a breakdown of bone tissue by the osteoclasts. These hormones are *estrogen* and *calcitonin*.

On the buildup side of bone formation are the osteoblasts, which make a glue-like protein called *collagen*. The collagen is woven into a type of matrix at the cites where the osteoclasts have etched cavities. Calcium and phosphorous which have been absorbed from the digestive tract enter the bloodstream and are used in the bone-building matrix as a hardening agent. The male hormone, testosterone, and the female hormone, progesterone, play influential roles in this building process.

Vitamin D plays a major role in assisting the absorption of calcium and phosphorous into the bloodstream from the intestines. Vitamin D must be converted into a biologically active form of Vitamin D before it can assist in the absorption of these minerals. As we age, our body's ability to convert regular Vitamin D into this biologically active form declines. As a result, blood levels of calcium begin to fall slightly. It is essential to life itself that calcium blood levels remain very constant. To counteract this fall in calcium blood levels, the parathyroid gland excretes a hormone called PTH. This hormone's responsibility is to remove calcium from bones or teeth to stabilize the blood levels of calcium. The net result is a deficit of calcium in your bones or teeth. This deficit continues year after year until your bones become honeycombed in appearance.

We can see that bones are very active tissues from the early growth years all the way into old age. We cannot afford to ignore them. They need constant attention if they are going to see us through to old age. The next question is, what can we do to help maintain the delicate balance of breakdown and buildup?

Excess Protein: The Main Cause

Everything I have written up to now about osteoporosis is mainstream scientific knowledge about the disease. In this section on protein, I am going to substantially deviate from the mainstream scientific knowledge regarding the severity of excess protein in the development of osteoporosis. All of the authorities on osteoporosis indicate that excess protein is a contributing factor to the disease, but many of them don't consider it the main cause. In fact, new emerging research is beginning to point out the tremendous impact excess protein has on the development of this disease.

Let's look at the ways excess protein affects our blood and bone calcium stores. I mentioned previously that the blood calcium levels are strictly controlled. One of the reasons for this involves the necessity of the blood to be at a certain "*pH*" level. The pH refers to the acidity or alkalinity of a substance. A pH of 7 is considered neutral. A pH of 0 is extremely acidic and a pH of 14 is extremely basic. The inner workings of your body are similar to a chemical processing plant. Numerous chemical reactions are always occurring. Some reactions produce a net base result and some produce an acidic result. Your blood must be maintained at a pH of approximately 7.2 - 7.3 at all times in order for your heart to beat properly, your muscles to contract, and your nervous system to function normally. Therefore, your body must perform a delicate balancing act with all these chemical reactions going on in order to maintain your blood at the proper pH.

Protein metabolism produces an acidic end result.

The more protein (especially animal protein) we consume, the higher the amount of acidic by-product the body will have to deal with in order to keep the blood at its proper pH. How does our body handle the acidic by-products of protein metabolism? The body uses, among other systems, the buffer salts of calcium and magnesium to help neutralize the strong acidic by-products of protein metabolism. Where does the body get the buffer salts? The calcium and magnesium needed to buffer the acidic effect of protein metabolism comes from your blood supply. Your blood supply is maintained from dietary sources of these minerals and your reserves in your bones and teeth.

Here's the catch: when your dietary intake of protein is too high, your blood must call on the reserves in your bones and teeth to maintain the balance it needs. When blood calcium levels fall to a certain level, your parathyroid gland excretes a hormone called PTH. The function of PTH is to cause a release of calcium from your bones and teeth into your blood stream to maintain proper blood levels of calcium at all times.

How much protein should we be eating? The U.S. Recommended Dietary Allowance (RDA) for adult women is 44 grams per day. The RDA for men is 56 grams per day. You must realize that there is a margin of safety built into this average, so your real need is probably 5 to 10 grams less.

The average American consumes almost three times this amount. When you consider that a cheeseburger has about 30 grams of protein; a 6 oz. sirloin about 46 grams; a glass of milk, 8 grams; and a 3 oz. piece of chicken light meat, 25 grams, -- you can see that we get our daily need for protein in one meal instead of three.

The RDA for calcium has just recently been increased because we are apparently loosing the battle with osteoporosis. The real problem is the fact that we con-

TOO MUCH PROTEIN

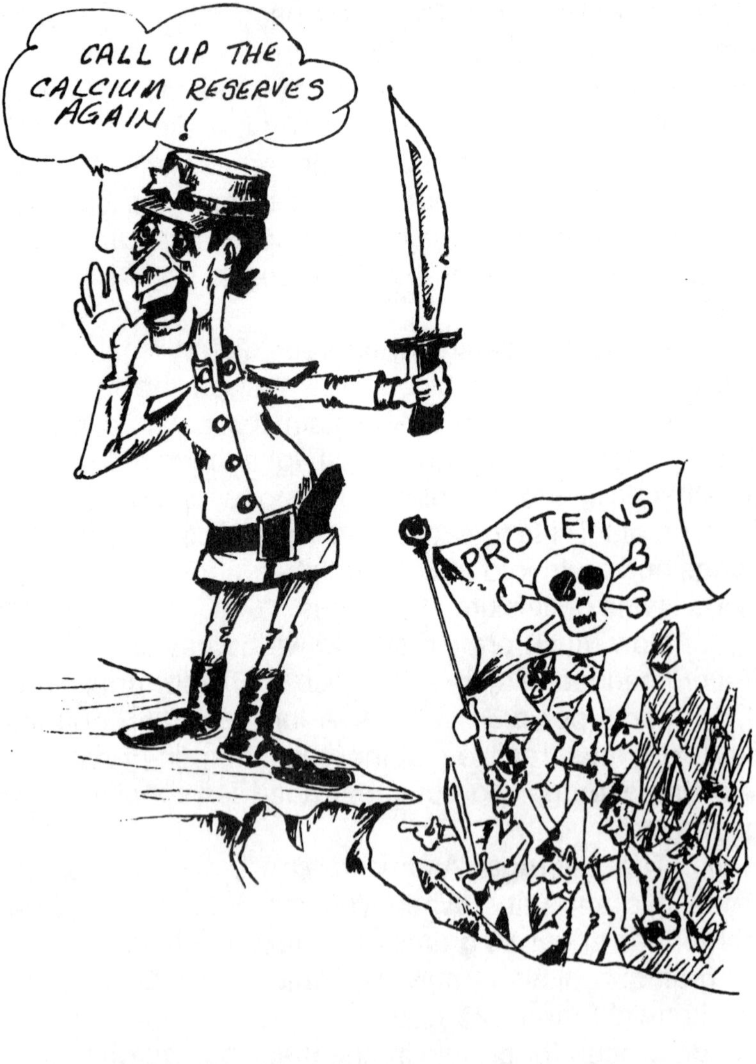

WASTES CALCIUM RESERVES

tinue to consume far more protein than our bodies can handle with the consequent use of our valuable bone calcium stores. We probably only need 400 to 600 hundred milligrams of calcium a day instead of the RDA of 800 to 1200 milligrams presently recommended. How can I make such a statement with all the so-called authorities recommending much more? I am a vigilant student of epidemiological studies from around the world. Populations in other parts of the world eat very differently than the industrialized countries of the world. As a consequence, they don't have the same diseases we do.

A study begun in China in 1983, led by T. Colin Campbell, Ph.D., of the Division of Nutritional Sciences at Cornell University, looked at the dietary habits of 6,500 Chinese. The differences in their eating habits correlated with the differences in types of diseases they developed. One striking difference is that the Chinese consume a third less protein than Americans do and, of that protein, they consume one-tenth as much protein from animal foods.[4]

The Chinese diet is mainly vegetarian, consisting of 77 percent complex carbohydrates derived from rice, grains, and vegetables. The Chinese diet has very little room for animal products. This type of diet also yields a very high fiber content. The Chinese, in many regions of their country, consume as much as 77 grams of fiber per day.[5] According to American scientists, both high-fiber diets and vegetarian diets can contribute to osteoporosis. The Chinese study has apparently proven them wrong. The incidence of osteoporosis in China is almost nonexistent.

High Dairy Consumption Is Not the Answer

Here is the big surprise that has come out of the

recent Chinese study and other similar studies from populations around the world. *The countries that have the highest intake of calcium from dairy products have the highest incidence of osteoporosis.* The United States is one of the largest consumers of dairy products in the world. It is no accident that the United States has one of the highest incidences of osteoporosis in the world. This recent information is in direct conflict with conventional wisdom on osteoporosis.

The main reason dairy products, such as milk and cheese, contribute to osteoporosis instead of retard it, is the fact that dairy products are very high in protein. Dairy milk is for calves not humans. I realize this is a very alarming statement, but the evidence from population studies is mounting to support what I have just said about dairy products.

A recent study conducted at the University of Texas has found that a predominately vegetarian diet has a protective effect against osteoporosis and that meat-based diets appear to be the cause of the disease.[6] Animal-based and plant-based diets have a different effect on the way the body metabolizes calcium. A diet high in animal-based proteins increases the amount of acid in the body. The bones then try to buffer the acid by releasing the calcium. The body then excretes the calcium, causing bone loss.[7] In the University of Texas study, the risk for developing osteoporosis progressively increased as the subject's diet is switched from vegan (no dairy products or eggs) to ovo-vegetarian (including eggs but no dairy products) to meat. "This study suggests that a diet higher in vegetable protein might actually be somewhat protective against osteoporosis," says Dr. Neil Breslau, one of the researchers.[8]

As more of these types of studies are conducted in the United States, I believe that, in the coming years, American scientists will rewrite their books on the role of dairy products in this disease and discover the real causes for this disease. In the meantime, we cannot afford to wait for conventional wisdom to catch up with the facts coming out of worldwide epidemiological studies today.

Reduce your protein consumption now to the RDA established for you. Look for alternative sources of dietary calcium such as broccoli and almonds. If you must supplement, do it wisely. Research has indicated that calcium is absorbed better in an acid environment. One good nondairy-supplemented source of calcium is ***Minute Maid*** Calcium Fortified Orange Juice. One eight-ounce glass of this orange juice has as much calcium as a glass of milk, without the high protein content.

Exercise and Osteoporosis

Of all the things we can do to strengthen our bones, exercise is one of the most important. Exercise acts on the bones the same way it acts on the muscles. When you lift weights, the muscles involved become bigger and stronger. Studies have shown that the bones involved with the muscles have also increased in size and density. More specifically, weight-bearing exercise increases the size and density of the bones which are involved in the exercise. Exercises such as walking, jogging, tennis, stair-climbing, and low impact aerobics have been shown in studies to increase the bone size and density of the participants.

Population studies from around the world indicate that people who lead more active, vigorous lifestyles have much less incidence of osteoporosis. Scientists have noticed for centuries that the bones in the arms of civilizations that hunt by throwing spears, bolas, or boomerangs have always been larger and more dense than other parts of the body. Galileo observed this connection way back in the seventeenth century. Modern research has concluded that every motion that you make affects how your bones are used in this motion. The type of motion or exercise you engage in, as well as how often you do so, influences the size and density of the bones you are using most in order to perform the exercise.[9]

How you use your bones affects their size and strength. Bone is very much like muscle," says Everett Smith, Ph.D., Director of the Biogerontology Laboratory at the University of Wisconsin. "If you exercise it, it gets bigger. If you stop, it atrophies. All you have to do is look at the forearm of a tennis player to see the effect of exercise. Not only is the muscle overdeveloped, but the bone is larger too." You know the old saying, "Use it, or lose it." It definitely applies to bones.

Exercise can slow down or retard the negative bone changes brought about by osteoporosis. A 3-year study conducted on elderly women in their eighties who engaged in regular weight-bearing exercise 3 days a week showed significant increases in their bone mineral content.[10]

We have all been told about the benefits of a regular exercise program. We now know that the ***type*** of exercise can influence other aspects of your health. Everyone should include some form of weight-bearing exercise into their weekly regimen for the health of their bones. Weight-bearing or resistance-type exercises, such as isometrics, help the bones in several ways. First, lifting weights or doing isometrics increases the strength of the muscles you use. This increase in strength will in itself protect the bones and joints from sudden jars or jolts resulting from wrenching motions or a fall. The stronger and denser the muscle, the more stress and impact it can absorb.

Secondly, research indicates that the act of lifting a weight puts a stress not only on the muscles affected, but also on the bones affected. In order for strength and growth to occur, stress must be placed on the muscle or bone. Analysis of professional weight lifters' bone densities indicate much stronger, denser bones than the average population. The double protection ability of stronger muscles and denser bones makes weight-lifting exercises ideal for your maximum bone-strengthening program.

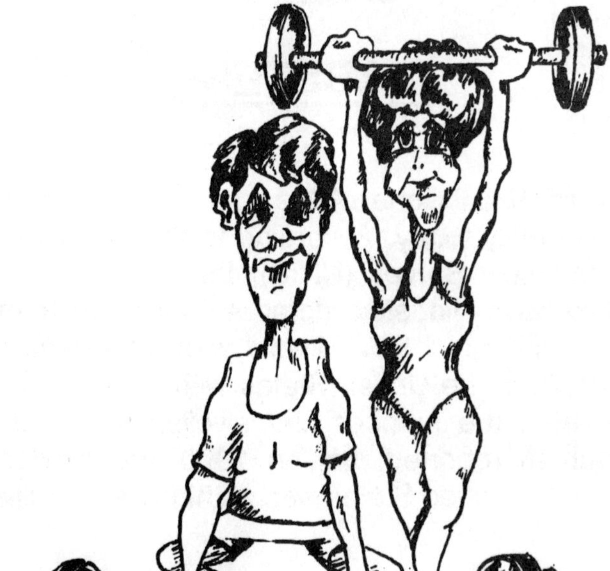

Chapter 8

DIABETES

DIABETES is one of the four major deterrents to longevity today. According to the National Health Interview Survey (NHIS), the number of people reported to have diabetes increased by more than 17% from 1980 through 1987. There was an estimated 5.8 million people in the United States with diabetes in 1980, and, by 1987, the number had swollen to 6.8 million.[1] Other sources reported that, in 1990, the incidence of diabetes in the United States was as high as 11 million.[2]

What is Diabetes?

Diabetes is the loss of the body's ability to utilize dietary sources of glucose due to little or no insulin production, or reduced sensitivity of cells to insulin. Basically, glucose is unable to get into the cells. When this occurs, glucose builds up in the blood. It is the job of the kidneys to retain glucose, but when the glucose levels become too high, the kidneys release it into the urine. The presence of glucose in the urine is one of the tests for diabetes.

The function of insulin is to help the body regulate and store glucose (sugar). Glucose is the body's main source of energy. Blood levels of glucose must be regulated strictly to provide a ready source of energy for the brain and nervous system. Insulin provides this regulation. Insulin also directs the storage of glucose into the liver and muscles. Dietary intake of carbohydrates, fats, and proteins are the body's source of glucose.

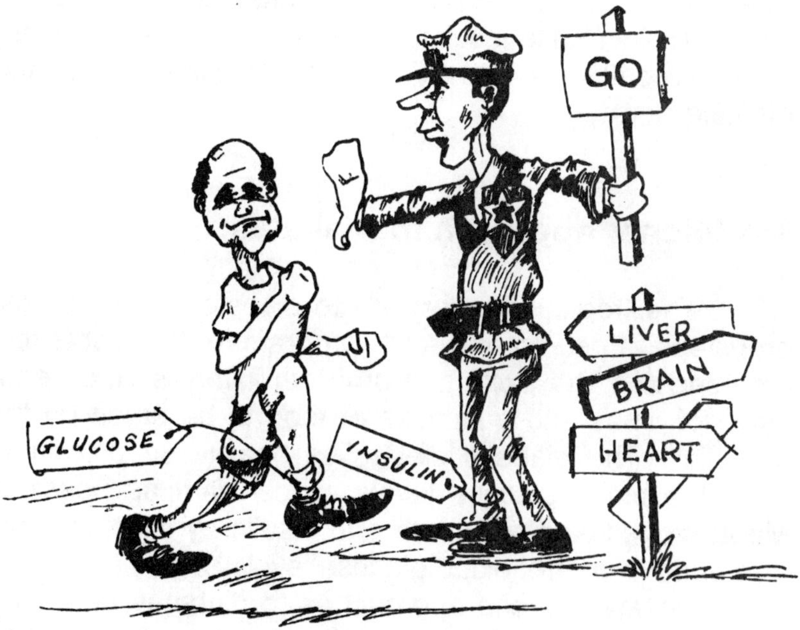

There are two prevalent types of diabetes: *insulin-dependent* and *noninsulin-dependent.* Insulin-dependent diabetes is also called juvenile/child-onset diabetes, usually starting in childhood with little or no production of insulin. This is the most severe form of diabetes, often occurring after a viral infection which destroys the cells of the pancreas responsible for the production of insulin. After these cells are destroyed, the victim of this disease must take insulin for the rest of his or her life. Juvenile/child diabetes accounts for only about 7% of the total incidence of diabetes in the United States.[3] Noninsulin-dependent diabetes, or adult-onset diabetes, is the most prevalent and controllable type of diabetes. Adult- onset diabetes accounts for about 97% of the incidence of the disease in the United States.[4] This form of the disease does not have the problem of too little insulin, but of the cells inability to use insulin. Weight gain and a sedentary lifestyle contribute heavily to the development of this disease.

Traditional Approach to Diabetes

The traditional approach to diabetes involves several steps. First, an exchange program for the diet is recommended. The exchange program involves strict regulation of types and quantities of food to be eaten by the diabetic. The diabetic diet relies heavily on protein to keep the blood glucose levels as constant as possible. Medications taken by mouth and insulin by injections are also used to control blood glucose levels.

However, these approaches to diabetes only control one aspect of diabetes: the blood glucose levels. The disease affects many other systems of the body as well. Most diabetics suffer blindness, heart attacks or kidney failure within 17 years after diagnosis of the disease.[5]

Even if you take insulin or other medications to lower your blood glucose levels, the damage to blood vessels will continue unchecked. Taking medication to control blood glucose levels increases the risk of dying from heart disease by 2-1/2 times more than that of diabetics controlling their glucose levels by diet alone.[6]

Better Strategies for Controlling Diabetes

Like many of the other diseases associated with prosperity, diabetes is most prevalent among industrialized nations which practice diets high in fat and low in fiber.

Diet

Diet can play a major role in the control of diabetes. A low-fat, low-protein, high-complex carbohydrate diet is the main solution to controlling diabetes. The American Diabetic Association has recently changed its stance on the role of carbohydrates in the diabetic's diet. Its new recommendations increase the recommended percentage of carbohydrates in the diabetic's diet from 45% to 65%. This new recommendation reflects current knowledge of carbohydrates' ability to stimulate insulin activity. Fat has been shown to block the effects of insulin. Eating a low-fat diet will solve this part of the problem. Low-fiber diets allow glucose to leave the intestines too rapidly. A high-fiber diet slows the release of glucose from the intestines into the blood. This slow release of glucose helps maintain a steady blood glucose level.

Diabetes puts a strain on many organs of the body. One organ especially burdened by diabetes is the kidney. High-protein diets cause the kidneys to work overtime in eliminating many of the toxic by-products of its digestion.

Lowering the protein content of the diabetic's diet lessens the burden of the already overworked kidneys.

The food we eat is broken down into the primary energy source: glucose. As glucose enters the bloodstream, insulin is secreted from the pancreas. The function of insulin is to assist the cells in the storage of glucose, amino acids, and fatty acids. The problem in adult-onset diabetes is that the insulin receptors on the cells' surface have become desensitized and inefficient. One of the consequences of the inefficient insulin cell receptors is an improper use of the blood glucose. Since the insulin receptors are not functioning properly, the blood glucose levels fluctuate up and down in an uncontrolled manner.

Exercise

Exercise is another factor very beneficial for the diabetic. A new study in *The New England Journal of Medicine* confirms that exercise may actually prevent diabetes. The researchers found that middle-aged men who exercise regularly lowered their chance of developing adult-onset diabetes by 6% for every 500 calories burned per week.[7] Exercise helps the body control blood glucose levels. Exercise builds strong hearts and helps lower body fat. One side effect of diabetes is less circulation to the extremities. Exercise helps to increase the blood flow to all parts of the body, including the extremities. Exercise can also lower levels of circulating blood fats. These blood fats, in the form of cholesterol and triglycerides, block the action of insulin. There is also some evidence that exercise increases the number of insulin receptors on cell surfaces, which means insulin can find a place to put glucose, and glucose can get to where it's needed inside the cells.[8] **Before engaging in an exercise program, inform your doctor.** Your doctor will need to help you regulate any medication you may be taking as the exercise program begins to lower your glucose levels.

The liver is one of the main storage places where glucose is deposited. Another main storage area for glucose is in the muscles. It is insulin's job to direct blood glucose to be stored in one of these two main sights. Muscle cells are the site of major insulin resistance when diabetes occurs.[9] Muscle cells normally store glucose with the aid of insulin in the form of glycogen for future use during activities involving the muscles.

When diabetes occurs, the insulin receptors on the muscle cells' surface are resistant to the storage of glucose. If the muscle cells refuse the glucose, it must go somewhere else. The glucose is then stored as fat. The irony of this is that fat in the blood and fat cells themselves generally hinder insulin's effectiveness. As the muscle cells reject the glucose, and the glucose is forced to be stored as fat, a vicious cycle develops. Exercise can dismantle the stages of this cycle. Once you start to lose weight from an exercise program, the fat cells begin to shrink in size. When you become more efficient at storing glucose in the muscles instead of as fat, the whole body begins to lean out, thus breaking the vicious cycle.

The major cause of the severe complications associated with diabetes is the body's need for external supplies of insulin to be injected into the blood. When diabetes is controlled without the help of external insulin, the complications are less severe. The stabilizing effect on the blood glucose levels and the increase in insulin receptors caused by exercise can, in most cases, entirely eliminate the need for external insulin.

The main goal of the diabetic should be to reduce medications of all kinds as much as possible. Medications only control one aspect of diabetes. There are many adverse effects of the disease which continue their damage even when the diabetic is on medication. If the diabetic can control blood glucose levels by diet and exercise without the use of medication, he or she will eliminate many of the other side affects of the disease.

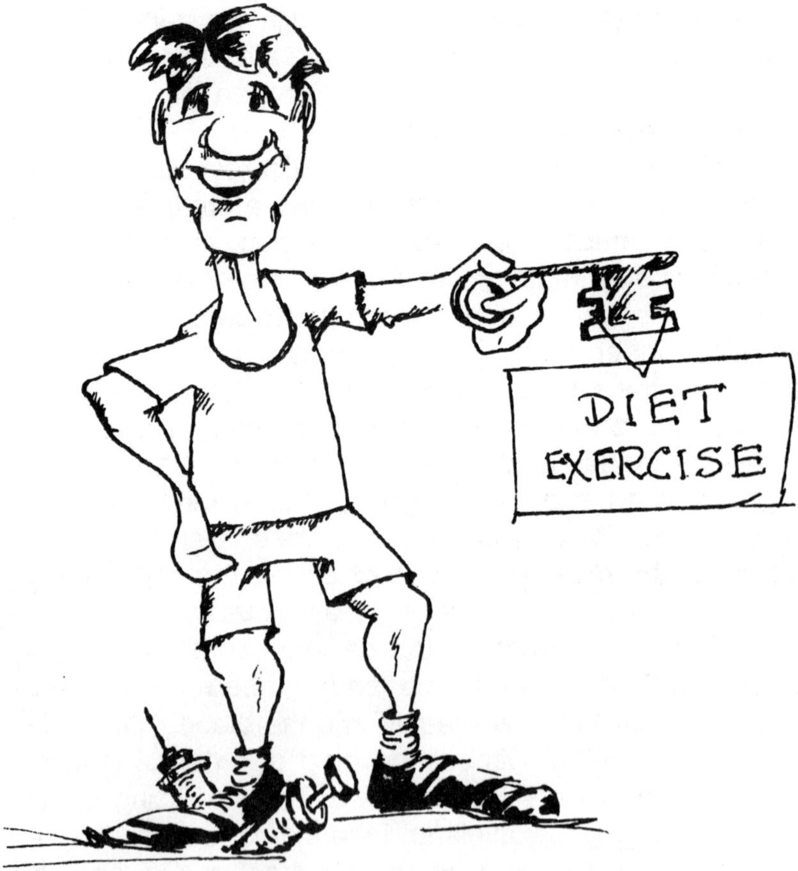

DIET AND EXERCISE ARE THE KEY

Chapter 9

IN THE BALANCE

IN the fast-paced society we live in today, everybody is looking for instant results. We've gotten used to instant meals (fast food restaurants, instant foods on the grocery shelf, microwavable items, etc.), instant service (have you noticed how popular drive-thrus have become?), instant credit, instant lotteries, instant energy boosts (ie, coffee, pep pills, sugar highs), instant gratification, instant marriages -- instant just-about-anything-you-want! We're so spoiled that we protest if we have to wait in line for something more than a minute. Is it any wonder than Americans expect instant health and slenderness plans?

If you've been loading your system with junk food for the past 40 years, have never bothered to exercise, have neglected to drink much water or get much rest, and have basically lived most of your life in bad health habits, why should you expect to suddenly glow with fitness after one or two weeks of some "fix-me-up-quick" diet or exercise scheme? Let's get realistic. You didn't get out of shape overnight, so give yourself a little time to get *in* shape. But listen, the encouraging news is that our bodies are able to respond remarkably fast to improved care! While you may not be able to see a 100% turnaround overnight if you're desperately out of shape, you *will* show signs of dramatic improvement very quickly when you change your bad habits into good ones. Our bodies are much more resistant to abuse than to tender loving care. In other words, it takes much more time for our bodies to show the signs of neglect than it does to evidence the signs of good treatment. Lung cancer due to cigarette smoking, for instance, doesn't develop right away. Our bodies actually tolerate a great deal of abuse before giving way. The results of proper toning exercises can sometimes be noticed within a matter of days. That doesn't mean that you'll necessarily be ready to model in a beauty contest in the first week, but you should see a change in your muscle tone if you've been diligently exercising the correct way. In the same way, it shouldn't take long for you to notice a change in your weight and appearance, as well as your level of energy and alertness, after sticking with the Lifetime Diet plan I've outlined in the previous chapter on weight loss.

Our bodies are much more resistant to abuse than to tender loving care...

Nonetheless, if we really want to increase our chances for a longer, healthier life, we need to get in touch with the total way of life we were designed for, rather than looking for one quick-fix solution after another. Total health requires a ***balance*** of all the things I've mentioned in this book. This means you need to pay attention to every aspect of who you are in body, mind and spirit. If you neglect any one of these aspects of your personhood, you will eventually suffer the unpleasant consequences. I say "eventually" because you may not notice right away. You might even convince yourself that you're "in balance." But if you're not really in balance, it will show up sooner or later.

Maybe you're slender like the student I mentioned in Chapter 5 who ate all kinds of junk food and never gained an ounce. So maybe the consequences of your poor eating habits aren't evident yet, but what about ten years down the road? Is it really worth the risk? Or maybe you're like Lou who led an "active" lifestyle and looked fit enough on the outside, until his poor eating habits caught up with him later in life and resulted in heart disease. Too many people don't think about the future consequences of current bad habits, and stories abound of how their bad habits eventually caught up with them. Or maybe you do take good care of your body. You exercise, drink plenty of fresh water, get enough rest, eat the right foods, nourish your skin, and basically do all the right things for your body. So your body is in good shape. But what if you then start leading a promiscuous lifestyle. Who's to say you won't eventually get AIDS or some other Sexually Transmitted Disease? Wouldn't it be a shame to see such a beautiful body waste away with AIDS? No matter how diligently you follow the rules for proper physical care of your body, if you neglect the rules for proper spiritual (moral) health, it will ultimately affect your body.

Or perhaps you live a moral lifestyle. Maybe you even have a relationship with God and are spiritually fulfilled in that relationship. But if you neglect your body, don't expect God to keep "fixing" the damage you keep doing over and over to yourself. It's not that He can't fix it, but He's given you principles to follow, and these principles happen to include instructions about caring for our bodies. He wants you to understand these instructions and obey them. If you don't, you may just have to suffer some natural consequences.

Then there's the emotional imbalance so many of us suffer -- sometimes without even being aware of it. Maybe you are nourishing your body and spirit with the right things, but you are harboring hatred, bitterness, fear, or anxiety in your heart. If you don't deal with these feelings, they will eventually destroy you. Bitterness doesn't hurt the person we're bitter toward. It hurts the one who's harboring the bitterness. It's like an acid that eats away at your insides, often resulting in ulcers, gastric disorders, headaches or heart failure. It also eats away at relationships and soon begins to affect every aspect of our lives. Bitterness can be a very destructive force.

And as for the results of an intellectual imbalance, consider this. If you fail to educate your mind, how are you going to even *know* how to take care of the rest of you?

It is essential to stay in balance?

Another aspect of staying in balance has to do with moderation versus excess. Too much of a good thing can become a destructive thing. Fire can be a good thing in the right balance. It takes fire to start the engine of a car. It takes fire to cook with and fire to create heat for our homes and light for a dark place. But fire out of control is destructive. Wine can be good in moderation, but destructive in excess. The Bible says that honey is good, but too much honey makes one sick (Proverbs 25:16). Do you remember how I demonstrated in Chapter Two that some measure of lipids (fats), as in cholesterol, are necessary in our system for proper functioning? And do you remember how I told you that it's not the fats themselves that are the bad guys, but it's when they overpopulate that problems arise? Moderation is an important key to the door which helps keep us in balance. But the exciting thing about my Lifetime Diet Plan is that it takes more than any normal person could eat to get past the "moderation" point regarding the foods in this diet. You should be able to eat as much as you like without negative consequences. You should never have to go hungry again if you eat enough of the right foods. And if you combine this diet with the right exercises, plenty of water, rest, fresh air, a positive attitude, and a wholesome balance of body, soul and spirit, you will feel better than you ever thought you could.

If you follow the Lifetime Plan I've outlined in this book, and keep your life in better balance, you can not only increase your natural life span by twenty or more years, but can improve your whole well-being. Your physical appearance will improve. Not only will your weight balance out to where it should be, but even your skin and hair will improve. Your energy level will increase, your appetite will become healthier in the respect of craving the right foods instead of the bad ones, and you will discover more stamina, clarity of thought, and a more joyful spirit.

Well, I've done my part in telling you about this exciting way to live. Now the rest is up to you. Do you want a longer, healthier life? If you've read this far, you probably do. If so, then do something about it. The key's in your hand. How are you going to use it? Keep in mind that, if you choose to follow only part of the Lifetime Plan I've outlined, you cannot enjoy the full benefits of the total plan. The earlier you get started on the Lifetime Plan, the better. But it's never too late.

So, here's to you and your 120th birthday celebration!

The Lifetime Diet Guide

In the following pages, I have developed 2 different types of tables. The first table is for those of you who know that you cannot realistically give up all your fast foods overnight. I have therefore listed some popular fast food choices for you to pick from when you do succumb to such foods. These Fast Food Tables will help you recognize just what you are putting into your mouth when you eat at a fast food restaurant. I have rated the value of such foods according to the amount of fat, sodium, and calories in each, and have given them a final rating from 1 to 6, with "1" being the best choice and "6" being the worst.

Some interesting facts will emerge when you start to study some of these tables. Did you know, for instance, that not all chicken sandwiches are created equal? Take a look at the fat content of some of the different chicken sandwiches listed in my Fast Food Sandwich Guide. You will see a significant difference between the best and worst sandwiches.

I call the next set of tables "Smart Food Tables." This is a guide which rates the smarter food choices. These are the foods you need to aim for as much as possible.

After these tables is a 12-day sample diet plan for you to follow, including recipes and food value charts. I have tried to take the work out of hunting through food value tables to find the right foods to eat.

I hope these guides will be of some value to you in analyzing your diet and helping you make the necessary changes toward maximum health.

FAST FOOD

TABLES

(most of the data was provided by the individual food chains)

FAST FOOD BREAKFAST CHOICES

DESCRIPTION	CALORIES	FAT (gm)	SODIUM (mg)	RATING
ARBY'S ®				1 = Best 6 = Worst
Blueberry Muffin	200	6	269	3
Biscuit, Plain	280	15	730	4
Croissant, Plain	260	16	300	4
Biscuit, Ham	323	17	1169	5
Biscuit, Bacon	318	18	904	5
Croissant, Ham & Cheese	345	21	939	6
Egg Platter	460	24	591	5
Croissant, Bacon & Egg	389	26	582	6
Biscuit, Sausage	460	32	1000	5
Croissant Mushrm Cheese	493	38	935	5
BURGER KING ®				
Croissant Plain	180	10	285	4
Mini Muffins, Blueberry	292	14	244	4
Croissan ' Wich Egg Chees	315	20	607	5
Croissan' Wich Ham Eg Ch	346	21	962	6
Croissan' Wich Bac Eg Ch	361	24	227	6
Croissan' Wich Sas Eg Ch	534	40	985	6
HARDEES ®				
Biscuit Ham	320	16	1000	6
Biscuit Cinnamon Raisin	324	17	510	5
Muffin Oat Bran Raisin	440	18	350	5
Biscuit Rise 'N' Shine	320	19	740	5
Biscuit Country Ham	350	21	1550	6
Muffin Blueberry	400	22	320	5
Biscuit Ham Eg	370	23	1050	6
Biscuit Bacon	360	24	950	6
Biscuit Cntry Ham Eg	400	27	1600	6
Biscuit Ham Eg Chees	420	28	1270	6
Biscuit Bacon Eg	410	29	990	6
Biscuit Canad Rise 'N' Sh	470	31	1550	6
Biscuit Sausage	440	32	1100	6
Biscuit Bacon Eg Cheese	460	28	1200	

FAST FOOD BREAKFAST CHOICES

DESCRIPTION	CALORIES	FAT (gm)	SODIUM (mg)	RATING
HARDEE'S ® (Cont'd)				1 = Best 6 = Worst
Biscuit Sausage & Egg	490	31	1150	6
Biscuit Steak & Egg	550	32	1370	6
McDONALD'S ®				
Muffin, Apple Bran Fat Free	180	0	200	3
Muffin, Blueberry Fat Free	170	0	220	2
English Muffin/Margarine	170	5	230	4
Mcmuffin, Egg	280	11	710	5
Biscuit With Brkfst Spread	260	13	730	5
Breakfast Burrito	280	17	580	5
Mcmuffin, Sausage	345	20	770	6
Mcmuffin, Sausage & Egg	415	25	915	6
Biscuit/ Bacon Egg Cheese	430	26	1190	6
Biscuit With Sausage	420	28	1040	6
Biscuit/ Sausage & Egg	500	33	1210	6

FAST FOOD SANDWICH CHOICES

DESCRIPTION	CALORIES	FAT (gm)	SODIUM (mg)	RATING
ARBY'S ®				1 = Best 6 = Worst
Light Roast Turkey Deluxe	249	4	1172	3
Light Roast Beef Deluxe	296	10	826	4
Roast Beef, Junior	218	11	345	5
French Dip Roast Beef	345	12	6787	4
Roast Beef, Regular	353	15	588	5
French Dip'n Swiss	425	18	1078	5
Turkey Deluxe	399	20	1047	5
Beef'n Cheddar	451	20	955	5
Philly Beef'n Swiss	498	26	1194	5
Chicken Breast Sandwich	489	26	1019	5
Roast Beef, Giant	530	27	908	5
Roast Beef, Super	529	28	798	5
Fish Fillet Sandwich	537	29	994	5
Bac'n Cheddar Deluxe	532	33	1672	5
BURGER KING ®				
Bk Broiler Chicken	267	8	728	4
Hamburger	272	11	505	5
Cheeseburger	318	15	661	5
Burger Buddies	349	17	717	6
Hamburger Deluxe	344	19	496	6
Cheeseburger Deluxe	390	23	652	6
Ocean Catch Fish Fillet	495	25	879	6
Double Cheeseburger	483	27	851	5
Bacon Double Cheese	515	31	748	6
Whopper	614	36	865	6
Bacon Double Cheese Dlx	592	39	804	6
Chicken Sandwich, Fried	685	40	1417	6
Whopper With Cheese	706	44	1177	6
Whopper, Double	844	53	933	6
Whopper, Double, Cheese	935	61	125	6
HARDEE'S ®				
Grilled Chicken	310	9	890	4
Hamburger	270	10	490	5

FAST FOOD SANDWICH CHOICES

DESCRIPTION	CALORIES	FAT (gm)	SODIUM (mg)	RATING
HARDEE'S ® (CONT'd)				1 Best 6 Worst
Roast Beef Sandwich	350	11	732	4
Real Lean Deluxe	340	13	650	4
Cheeseburger	320	14	710	5
Roast Beef Big	360	15	1150	4
Roast Beef With Cheese	403	15	954	5
Turkey Club	390	16	1280	5
Fisherman's Fillet	500	24	1030	6
Big Twin	450	25	580	6
Mushroom N' Swiss	490	27	940	5
Quarter Pnd Cheeseburger	500	29	1060	6
Big Deluxe Burger	500	30	760	6
Bacon Cheeseburger	610	39	1030	6
McDONALD'S ®				
Grilled Chicken Sandwich	252	4	740	3
Chicken Fajitas	185	8	310	4
Hamburger	255	9	490	5
Mclean Deluxe	320	10	670	5
Cheeseburger	305	13	710	5
Mclean Deluxe /Cheese	370	14	890	5
Filet-o-Fish	370	18	930	6
McChicken	415	20	770	6
Quarter Pounder	410	20	650	6
Big Mac	500	26	890	6
Quarter Pounder/Cheese	510	28	1090	6
SUBWAY (6") ®				
Sandwich, Turkey	357	10	839	4
Sandwich, Ham	360	11	839	5
Sandwich, Roast Beef	375	11	839	4
Sandwich, Subway club	379	11	839	4
Sandwich, Seafood/Crab	388	12	1306	4
Sandwich, Tuna	402	13	905	5
Sandwich, Meatball	429	16	876	5

(continued next page)

FAST FOOD SANDWICH CHOICES

DESCRIPTION	CALORIES	FAT (gm)	SODIUM (mg)	RATING
TACO BELL ®				1 = Best 6 = Worst
Tostada Fiesta	167	7	324	4
Taco Soft Fiesta	147	7	361	4
Taco Fiesta Beef	127	7	139	4
Pinto's & Cheese	190	9	642	4
Taco Chicken Hard Shell	171	9	337	4
Burrito Fiesta	226	9	652	4
Taco Hard Shell Beef	183	11	276	5
Taco Shoft Steak	218	11	456	5
Tostada Beef/Red Sauce	243	11	596	4
Burrito Chicken/No Sauce	334	12	880	5
Taco Soft Beef	225	12	554	5
Burrito Bean/Red Sauce	447	14	1148	5
Tostada Chicken/Sauce	264	15	454	5
Taco Supreme	230	15	276	5
Burrito Combination	407	16	1136	5
Taco Supreme Soft	272	16	554	5
Nachos	346	18	399	5
Burrito Beef/Red Sauce	493	21	1311	6
Burrito Suprem/Red Sauce	503	22	1181	6
Taco Bellgrande	335	23	472	6
Nachos Supreme	367	27	471	6
Nachos bellgrande	649	35	997	6
WENDY'S ®				
Grilled Chicken Sandwich	320	9	715	4
JR. Hamburger	260	9	570	4
Hamburger Single	340	15	500	5
JR. Swiss Deluxe	360	18	765	5
Chicken Sandwich Fried	430	19	725	6
Cheeseburger	410	21	760	5
Hamburger Singel/Every	420	21	890	6
Fish Filet Sandwich	460	25	780	6
Hamburger Double	520	27	710	6
Chicken Club Sandwich	506	28	930	6
JR. Bacon Cheeseburger	430	28	835	6
Big Classic	640	29	1345	6
Big Classic Double	750	45	1295	6

FAST FOOD CHICKEN & TURKEY

DESCRIPTION	CALORIES	FAT (gm)	SODIUM (mg)	RATING
ARBY'S ®				1 = Best 6 = Worst
Light Roast Turkey Deluxe	249	4	1172	3
Light Roast Chicken Dlx	253	5	874	3
Chicken Fajita Pita	256	9	787	4
Grilled Chicken Barbequ	378	14	1059	4
Roast Chicken Deluxe	373	19	913	5
Turkey Deluxe	399	20	1047	5
Grilled Chicken Deluxe	426	21	877	5
Chicken Breast Sandwich	489	26	1019	5
Roast Chicken Club	513	29	1423	5
BURGER KING ®				
Bk Broiler Chicken	267	8	728	4
Chicken Tenders 6 pcs	236	13	541	6
Chicken Sandwich, Fried	685	40	1417	6
HARDEE'S ®				
Grilled Chicken	310	9	890	4
Chicken 6 pcs	210	9	680	6
Chicken Fillet	370	13	1060	5
Turkey Club	390	16	1280	5
Biscuit Chicken	430	22	1330	5
McDONALD'S ®				
Grilled Chkn Brst Sandwich	252	4	740	3
Chicken Fajitas	185	8	310	4
Chicken Mcnuggets 6 pcs	270	15	580	6
McChicken	415	20	770	6
SUBWAY®				
Sandwich Turkey 6"	357	10	839	4

(continued next page)

FAST FOOD CHICKEN & TURKEY

DESCRIPTION	CALORIES	FAT (gm)	SODIUM (mg)	RATING
TACO BELL ®				1 = Best 6 = Worst
Meximelt Chicken	257	15	779	5
Tostada Chicken/Sauce	264	15	454	5
WENDY'S ®				
Grilled Chicken Sandwich	320	9	715	4
Chicken Sandwich Fried	430	19	725	6
Crispy Chicken Nuggets	280	20	600	6
Chicken Club Sandwich	506	28	930	6
KENTUCKY FRIED CHICKEN ®				
Original Recipe Drumstick	146	8	275	6
Chicken Littles Sandwich	169	10	331	6
Original Recipe Wing	178	12	372	6
Extra Tasty Crispy Drmstk	204	14	324	6
Original Recipe cntr Breast	283	15	672	6
Kentucky Nuggets 6 pcs	276	17	677	6
Extra Tast Crispy Wing	254	19	688	6
Hot Wings 6 pcs	372	24	677	6
Colonel's Chkn Sandwich	482	27	1060	6
Deluxe Chkn Sandwich	547	32	1362	6

FAST FOOD PIZZA

DESCRIPTION	CALORIES	FAT (gm)	SODIUM (mg)	RATING
DOMINO'S PIZZA ® (2 SLICES)				**1 = Best 6 = Worst**
Cheese , Thin	376	10	483	4
Ham, Thin	417	11	805	5
Sausage Mushroom, Reg	430	16	552	6
Pepperoni ,Thin	460	17	825	6
Veggie, Reg	498	18	1035	4
Deluxe, Thin	498	20	954	6
Double Cheese Peprni	545	25	1042	6
PIZZA HUT ® (2 SLICES)				
Thin'n Crispy Med	398	17	867	4
Pan Cheese Med	492	18	34	4
Trad Hand Tos Ches Med	518	20	1276	5
Thin'n Crspy Pep Med	413	20	986	6
Thin'n Crspy Sup Supr Med	463	21	1336	6
Pan Pepp eroni Med	540	22	1127	6
Trad Hand Tos Pepp Med	500	23	1267	6
Pan Super Supreme Med	563	26	1447	6
Trad Hand Tos Supr Med	540	26	1470	6
Personal Pan Supr Whole	647	28	1313	6
Personal Pan Pepp Whole	675	29	1335	6
Pan Supreme Med	589	30	1363	6
TACO BELL ®				
Mexican Pizza Whole	575	37	1031	6

FAST FOOD
POTATOES & FRENCH FRIES

DESCRIPTION	CALORIES	FAT (gm)	SODIUM (mg)	RATING
ARBY'S ®				1 = Best 6 = Worst
Plain Baked	240	1	58	1
Pototato Cake	204	12	397	6
French Fries, Small	246	13	114	6
Curly Fries	337	18	591	6
Broccoli & Cheddar	417	18	351	3
French Fries, Medium	394	21	182	6
Cheddar Fries	399	22	443	6
Baked/Butter & Sour Crem	463	25	203	4
French Fries, Large	492	25	228	6
Baked Potato Deluxe	515	27	923	4
BURGER KING ®				
Tater Tenders	213	12	318	6
French Fries, Medium	372	20	238	6
HARDEE'S ®				
French Fries, Regular	230	11	85	6
Hash Rounds	230	14	560	6
Crispy Curls	300	16	840	6
French Fries, Large	360	17	135	6
French Fries "Big Fry"	500	23	180	6
McDONALD'S ®				
Hashbrown Potatoes	130	7	330	6
French Fries, Small	220	12	110	6
French Fries, Medium	320	17	150	6
French Fries Large	400	22	200	6
WENDY'S ®				
Baked Potato, Plain	270	1	0	1
French Fries, small	240	12	145	6
Baked Potato/Cheese	420	15	310	3
French Fries Biggie	449	22	271	6

FAST FOOD SALAD DRESSING

DESCRIPTION	CALORIES	FAT (gm)	SODIUM (mg)	RATING
ARBY'S ®				1 = Best 6 = Worst
Wght Watchers Italn 1 oz.	29	3	NA	4
Honey French 2 oz.	322	27	486	5
Thousand Island 2 oz.	298	29	493	5
Blue Cheese 2 oz..	295	31	489	5
Buttermilk Ranch 2 oz.	349	38	471	5
			762	
BURGER KING ®				
Low Cal Lite Ital 2 oz.	170	18	762	5
French 2 oz.	290	22	400	6
Thousand Island 2 oz.	290	26	403	6
Bleu Cheese 2 oz.	300	32	512	6
Oil & Vinegar 2 oz.	310	33	214	6
Ranch 2 oz.	350	37	316	6
HARDEE'S ®				
Low Cal French 2 oz.	130	5	480	4
Low Cal Italian 2 oz.	90	8	310	4
Thousand Island 2 oz.	250	15	930	5
Blue Cheese 2 oz.	210	18	790	5
House 2 oz.	290	29	510	5
McDONALD'S ®				
Lite Vingrette 2 oz.	48	2	240	3
French Reduced Cal 2 oz.	160	8	460	4
Bleu Cheese 2.5 oz.	250	20	750	6
Ranch 2 oz.	220	20	520	6
WENDY'S ®				
Reduced Cal Itln 4 Tbsp	100	9	700	4
Red Cal Bcn/Tmto 4 Tbsp	100	16	760	5
Golden Italian 4 Tbsp	180	16	1000	5
Celery Seed 4 Tbsp	280	18	260	5
Italian Caesar 4 Tbsp	320	36	560	6

SMART FOOD

TABLES

VITAMIN C SMART CHOICES

DESCRIPTION	QUANTITY	VITAMIN C (mg)	CALORIES	RATING
Foods Listed by Highest Vitamin C Per Serving				**1 = Best 6 = Worst**
Orange Juice, Fresh	1 Cup	125	115	1
Strawberries/Sliced	1 Cup	120	68	1
Cantaloupe	1/2 Large	115	96	1
Papaya, Raw	1/2 Large	112	78	1
Broccoli, Cooked	1 Cup	97	45	1
Brussels Sprouts, Cooked	1 Cup	97	65	1
Green Pepper, Sweet	1 Pod	95	18	1
Watermelon	2" by 10"	94	300	1
Grapefruit	1 Medium	91	37	1
Oysters, Raw	1 Cup	70	160	3
Orange, Fresh	1 Medium	70	60	1
Cauliflower, Cooked	1 Cup	69	30	1
Mango, Fresh	1 Medium	57	135	1
Parsley, Chopped	1 Cup	54	20	1
Asparagus, Cooked	1 Cup	50	44	1
Collards, Frozen	1 Cup	45	60	1
Cabbage, Shredded	1 Cup	42	16	1
Spinach, Cooked	1 Cup	40	40	1
Honeydew Melon, Fresh	1 Cup	32	45	1
Raspberries, Fresh	1 Cup	31	60	1
Blackberries, Fresh	1 Cup	30	74	1
Sweet Potato, Peeled	1 Medium	28	120	1
Baked Potato, /skin	1 Medium	26	220	1
Pineapple chunks, Fresh	1 Cup	24	76	1
Tomato, Raw	1 Medium	22	24	1

VITAMIN A SMART CHOICES

DESCRIPTION	QUANTITY	VITAMIN A (RE)	CALORIES	RATING
Foods Listed by Highest Vitamin A Per Serving				**1 = Best 6 = Worst**
Sweet Potato	1 Medium	2480	120	1
Carrot, Whole	1 whole	2025	31	1
Spinach, Cooked	1 Cup	1470	41	1
Butternut Squash	1 Cup	1430	83	1
Collards, Frozen	1 Cup	1017	60	1
Winter Squash	1 Cup	870	96	1
Cantaloupe	1/2 Large	865	96	1
Mango, Fresh	1 Medium	806	135	1
Green Onions, Chopped	1 Cup	500	26	1
Papaya, Raw	1/2 Large	408	78	1
Watermelon	2" by 10"	350	300	1
Tomatoes, Cooked	1 Cup	325	60	1
Parsley, Chopped	1 Cup	312	20	1
Apricot Halves, Dried	10	253	83	1
Broccoli, Cooked	1 Cup	222	45	1
Oysters, Raw	1 Cup	220	160	3
Asparagus, Cooked	1 Cup	150	44	1
Romaine Lettuce, Chopped	1 Cup	146	9	1
Tomato whole, Raw	1 Each	139	24	1
Green Beans	1 Cup	83	44	1
Summer Squash	1 Cup	52	36	1
Peach Fresh, Medium	1 Each	47	37	1
Zucchini Squash	1 Cup	43	29	1
Green Pepper, Sweet	1 Cup	39	18	1

HIGH FIBER SMART CHOICES

DESCRIPTION	QUANTITY	FIBER	CALORIES	RATING
Foods Listed by Highest Fiber Per Serving				**1 = Best 6 = Worst**
Figs, Dried	10 Each	24	480	1
Kidney Beans	1 Cup	20	230	1
Pinto Beans	1 Cup	19	265	1
Prunes	10 Each	13.5	200	1
Black Beans	1 Cup	15	190	1
Great Northern Beans	1 Cup	12.5	210	1
All Bran Cereal	1/2 Cup	12	105	1
Blackberries	1 Cup	10	80	1
Black Eyed Peas	1 Cup	10	190	1
Lentils	1 Cup	10	215	1
Apples, Dried	10 Each	9	150	1
Raspberries	1 Cup	9	60	1
Oatmeal	1 Cup	9	145	1
Garbonzo Beans	1 Cup	8.5	270	1
Dates	10 Each	7	230	1
Broccoli, Cooked	1 Cup	6.5	45	1
Apple, Whole	1 Each	4-6	80-120	1
Pears	1 Each	5	98	1
Raisins	1/2 Cup	5	215	1
Strawberries/Sliced	1 Cup	5	68	1
Watermelon	2" by 4	5	30	1
Brussel Sprouts	1 Cup	5	65	1
Baked Potato/skin	1 Each	4.5	220	1
Sweet Potato, Peeled	1 Each	4	120	1
Parsley, Chopped	1 Cup	4	20	1
Collards	1 Cup	4	60	1
Apricot Halves	10 Each	3.5	80	1
Mango, Whole	1 Medium	3	135	1
Orange, Whole	1 Medium	3	60	1
Pineapple, Chunks	1 Cup	3	76	1
Asparagus, Cooked	1 Cup	3	44	1

SUPER FOOD
SMART CHOICES

DESCRIPTION	QUANTITY	VITAMIN A (RE)	VITAMIN C (mg)	FIBER
All Foods Excel In 2 Or More Nutrient Categories				
Sweet Potato, Peeled	1 Medium	2480	28	4
Cantaloupe	1/2 Large	865	115	2.5
Broccoli	1 Cup	222	97	6.5
Carrot, Whole	1 Whole	2025	10	2
Papaya, Raw	1/2 Large	408	112	2.5
Brussel Sprouts	1 Cup	114	97	5
Strawberries/sliced	1 Cup	7	120	5
Mango, Fresh	1 Medium	806	57	3
Orange	1 Medium	27	70	3
Parsley, Chopped	1 Cup	312	54	4
Collards, Cooked	1 Cup	1017	45	4
Blackberries	1 Cup	24	30	10
Green Pepper	1 Pod	39	95	1.3
Watermelon	2" by 10"	350	94	5
Cauliflower	1 Cup	t	69	1.7
Asparagus, Cooked	1 Cup	150		3.2
These Foods Are High In Fiber, Iron And Zinc				
Garbanzo Beans	1 Cup			8.5
Great Northern Beans	1 Cup			12.5
Kidney Beans	1 Cup			20
Lentils	1 Cup			10
Pinto Beans	1 Cup			19
Black beans	1 Cup			15
Lima Beans	1 Cup			10

12 - DAY

FOOD PLAN

(An asterisk* signifies that a recipe is provided)

Day One

Breakfast
3/4 cup cereal, oat bran flakes
1/2 cup skim milk
3/4 cup grapefruit juice
2 slices mixed grain bread, toasted
1/2 tbs *Promise Extra Light ®* margarine
1/2 medium cantaloupe

Lunch
1 Stuffed Pita Sandwich*
1 medium apple , with skin

Snack
1/4 cup raisins

Dinner
1/4 recipe, Vegetable Casserole with Couscous Crust*
1 cup salad, w/lettuce, tomato, carrot, cucumber, green pepper
1 tbs salad dressing, *Ranch, no oil, Pritikin ®*
1/2 cup fruit salad
1 baked potato with skin
1/2 tbs of *Promise Extra Light ®* margarine

Nutritional Information per Day

Calories	1468	**Daily %**	
Fat	20 gm.	Fat	13%
Protein	38 gm.	Protein	10%
Carbohydrate	276 gm.	Carbohydrate	76%
Fiber	43 gm.		

Vitamins & Minerals

Iron	15 mg.	Vitamin A	3572 RE
Calcium	640 mg.	Vitamin C	356 mg.

Day Two

Breakfast
1-1/4 cup cereal, *Cheerios, General Mills ®*
1/2 cup skim milk
1 cup orange juice, fresh
1 english muffin, plain
1/2 tbs of margarine, *Promise Extra Light ®*

Lunch
2 slices of whole wheat bread
1 plum, raw
1-1/2 cup Bean Salad*

Dinner
2 cups Garden Vegetable Barley*
1 slices of whole wheat bread
1 cup salad, w/lettuce, tomato, carrot, cucumber, green pepper
1 tbs salad dressing, *Ranch, no oil, Pritikin ®*
3/4 cup Strawberry Sherbert*

Nutritional Information per Day

Calories	1391	**Daily %**	
Fat	26 gm.	Fat	17%
Protein	38 gm.	Protein	11%
Carbohydrate	251 gm.	Carbohydrate	72%
Fiber	34 gm.		

Vitamins & Minerals

Iron	18 mg.	Vitamin A	1909 RE
Calcium	669 mg.	Vitamin C	331 mg.

Day Three

Breakfast
2 cups oatmeal
1/2 cup skim milk
1 banana
1 cup grapefruit juice

Lunch
1-1/2 cups Macaroni Salad*
1 whole wheat pita pocket, 6"

Dinner
1/4 recipe of Eggplant Lasagna*
2 slices multi-grain bread
2 cups Spinach Salad*
1 cup of strawberries

Nutritional Information per Day

Calories	1340	**Daily %**	
Fat	23 gm.	Fat	15%
Protein	49 gm.	Protein	15%
Carbohydrate	231 gm.	Carbohydrate	69%
Fiber	34 gm.		

Vitamins & Minerals

Iron	14 mg.	Vitamin A	1492 RE
Calcium	813 mg.	Vitamin C	258 mg.

Day Four

Breakfast
3 waffles, whole wheat blueberry*
1 cup orange juice, fresh
2 tbs low cal pancake syrup

Lunch
1 cup Mushroom Pilaf Soup*
1 whole wheat pita pocket, 6"

Dinner
1/4 recipe, Vegetarian Chili with Rice*
1 cup salad, w/lettuce, tomato, carrot, cucumber, green peeper
1 tbs salad dressing , Ranch, no oil, no sodium, *Pritikin ®*
2 slices bread, mixed grain, toasted
1 cup Melon Salad*

Nutritional Information per Day

Calories	1448
Fat	20 gm.
Protein	46 gm.
Carbohydrate	268 gm.
Fiber	31 gm.

Daily %	
Fat	13%
Protein	13%
Carbohydrate	74%

Vitamins & Minerals

Iron	15 mg.	Vitamin A	1616 RE
Calcium	645 mg.	Vitamin C	232 mg.

Day Five

Breakfast
1 cup cereal, G*rape-Nuts, Post ®*
1 cup skim milk
1 cup orange juice, fresh
1 cup strawberries, raw

Lunch
1 cup Quick Vegetable Barley Soup*
2 slices bread, *Hi-Fibre, Monks ®*
1/2 tbs margarine, *Promise Extra Light ®*
1 cup salad, w/lettuce, tomato, carrot, cucumber, green peeper
1 tbs salad dressing , *creamy italian, no oil, no sodium, Pritikin ®*
1 apple, raw

Snack
7 prunes, dried, without pits

Dinner
1 cup brown rice
1 cup corn, cooked
1/2 cup carrots, cooked
1 baked potato with skin
1/2 tbs margarine, *Promise Extra Light ®*

Nutritional Information per Day

Calories	1700	**Daily %**	
Fat	14 gm.	Fat	8%
Protein	47 gm.	Protein	11%
Carbohydrate	340 gm.	Carbohydrate	80%
Fiber	50 gm.		

Vitamins & Minerals

Iron	14 mg.	Vitamin A	3289 RE
Calcium	628 mg.	Vitamin C	263 mg.

Day Six

Breakfast
1 cup orange juice, fresh
1/4 recipe Fruit Salad*

Lunch
1 slice mixed grain bread
7 apricots, dried
1/4 recipe Special Vegetable Salad*

Dinner
1-1/2 cups brown rice
1 cup salad, w/lettuce, tomato, carrot, cucumber, green peeper
1 tbs salad dressing , *Caesar, reduced calorie, Pritikin ®*
2 slices mixed grain bread
2 baked potatoes with skin
1/2 tbs margarine, *Promise Extra Light ®*

Nutritional Information per Day

Calories	1616	**Daily %**	
Fat	22 gm.	Fat	13%
Protein	30 gm.	Protein	7%
Carbohydrate	317 gm.	Carbohydrate	82%
Fiber	34 gm.		

Vitamins & Minerals

Iron	15 mg.	Vitamin A	1460 RE
Calcium	379 mg.	Vitamin C	273 mg.

Day Seven

Breakfast
2 bananas

Snack
1 bagel, whole wheat
1 cup orange juice, *Minute Maid, Calcium Fortified ®*

Lunch
1 cup chili, *Vegetarian w/beans, spicy, no salt, Health Valley ®*
1 pita pocket, whole wheat, 6"

Snack
7 prunes, dried

Dinner
1 cup green beans, cooked
2 cups brown rice
1/2 cup carrots

Nutritional Information per Day

			Daily %	
Calories	1531			
Fat	18 gm.		Fat	10%
Protein	47 gm.		Protein	12%
Carbohydrate	291 gm.		Carbohydrate	77%
Fiber	50 gm.			

Vitamins & Minerals

Iron	14 mg.	Vitamin A	2235 RE
Calcium	682 mg.	Vitamin C	171 mg.

Day Eight

Breakfast
1 cup cereal, *Amaranth Crunch w/Raisins, Health Valley ®*
1/2 cup skim milk
1 cup orange juice, *Minute Maid, Calcium Fortified ®*

Snack
1 pear, medium
1/2 cantaloupe, medium

Lunch
1 cup soup, *Minestrone, no salt, Health Valley ®*
1 whole wheat pita pocket 6"

Dinner
1/4 recipe Lemon Catfish in Foil*
1/2 cup broccoli
1/2 cup cauliflower
1 sweet baked sweet potato

Nutritional Information per Day

Calories	1426	**Daily %**	
Fat	23 gm.	Fat	15%
Protein	55 gm.	Protein	15%
Carbohydrate	246 gm.	Carbohydrate	69%
Fiber	37 gm.		

Vitamins & Minerals

Iron	11 mg.	Vitamin A	1509 RE
Calcium	973 mg.	Vitamin C	373 mg.

Day Nine

Breakfast
1/2 cantaloupe, medium
1 banana
1 cup orange juice, *Minute Maid, Calcium Fortified ®*

Lunch
1 carrot, raw
1 Vegetable Sandwich*

Dinner
1 *Pita Pizza**
2 ear corn
1 baked potato, w/skin

Snack
10 prunes, dried

Nutritional Information per Day

			Daily %
Calories	1589		
Fat	17 gm.	Fat	10%
Protein	54 gm.	Protein	14%
Carbohydrate	298 gm.	Carbohydrate	75%
Fiber	46 gm.		

Vitamins & Minerals

Iron	12 mg.	Vitamin A	3261 RE
Calcium	1272 mg.	Vitamin C	307 mg.

Day Ten

Breakfast
2 cups cereal, *Nutri-Grain Corn, Kellogg's ®*
1 cup skim milk
1/2 cup apple juice

Snack
1 papaya, raw

Lunch
1 cup salad, w/lettuce, tomato, carrot, cucumber, green pepper
1 tbs salad dressing, r*anch, no oil, Pritikin ®*
1 whole wheat pita pocket 6"
1/2 tbs of margarine, *Promise Extra Light ®*

Dinner
1/4 pound Boiled Shrimp*
2 cups Spinach Salad*
1/2 cup broccoli, cooked
1/2 tbs of margarine, *Promise Extra Light ®*
1 baked potato
3/4 cup Strawberry Sherbert*

Nutritional Information per Day

		Daily %	
Calories	1588		
Fat	16 gm.	Fat	9%
Protein	65 gm.	Protein	16%
Carbohydrate	294 gm.	Carbohydrate	74%
Fiber	41 gm.		

Vitamins & Minerals

Iron	16 mg.	Vitamin A	2724 RE
Calcium	1339 mg.	Vitamin C	603 mg.

Day Eleven

Breakfast
1 cup cereal, *Bran Flakes, Kellogg's ®*
1/2 cup skim milk
1 cup orange juice, *Minute Maid, Calcium Fortified ®*

Snack
1 apple, raw
1 banana, raw

Lunch
1/4 recipe Hummus Tahini*
1 carrot, raw

Dinner
1/4 recipe for Lentils and Rice*
1/2 cup broccoli, cooked with 1/2 ounce cheddar cheese topping

Nutritional Information per Day

		Daily %	
Calories	1340		
Fat	14 gm.	Fat	9%
Protein	46 gm.	Protein	14%
Carbohydrate	257 gm.	Carbohydrate	76%
Fiber	35 gm.		

Vitamins & Minerals

Iron	39 mg.	Vitamin A	2654 RE
Calcium	1065 mg.	Vitamin C	202 mg.

Day Twelve

Breakfast
1 cup orange juice, *Minute Maid, Calcium Fortified ®*

Snack
1 banana, raw

Lunch
1 Light Roast Turkey Deluxe, Arby's ®

Dinner
2 baked potato
1 tbs of margarine, *Promise Extra Light ®*
1/2 cup carrots, cooked
2 ears of corn
1/2 cup frozen yogurt, nonfat

Nutritional Information per Day

Calories	1575	**Daily %**	
Fat	14 gm.	Fat	8%
Protein	53 gm.	Protein	13%
Carbohydrate	309 gm.	Carbohydrate	79%
Fiber	34 gm.		

Vitamins & Minerals

Iron	9 mg.	Vitamin A	3973 RE
Calcium	793 mg.	Vitamin C	409 mg.

HEALTHFUL

RECIPES

Stuffed Pita Sandwich

Serves: 4

1 tbs mayonnaise, reduced calorie
1/2 tsp oregano
1 oz. swiss cheese, low fat
4 radishes, trimmed and thinly sliced
4 lettuce leaves
1 tomato, chopped
1 tbs vinegar, white wine
1/4 tsp paprika
1 carrot, raw
4 whole wheat pita pockets
1 cup alfalfa sprouts

Instructions

1. Blend mayonnaise, vinegar, oregano and paprika in a medium sized bowl.
2. Stir in cheese, carrot and radishes.
3. Split open the pita pockets and insert a lettuce leaf in each.
4. Spoon the cheese/vegetable mixture over the lettuce.
5. Top with tomatoes and alfalfa sprouts

Nutritional Information per Serving

Calories	212	Carbohydrates	33 gm
Protein	9 gm	Fat	5 gm
Fiber	6 gm		

Vitamins & Minerals

Iron	2 mg	Vitamin A	574 RE
Calcium	141 mg	Vitamin C	10 mg

Vegetable Casserole with Couscous Crust

Serves: 4

1-1/2 cup chicken broth	1 cup couscous, prepared without fat
2 cups tomatoes, chopped	3/4 cup onions, raw
4 mushrooms, raw, whole	1 pepper,red, sweet
2 cups summer squash, sliced	2 carrots, raw
1 cup broccoli	1/2 cup garbanzo beans, cooked
1-1/2 tsp dried basil, crumbled	1/4 tsp black pepper

Instructions

1. Preheat oven to 350 degrees
2. In a medium saucepan over moderately high heat, bring chicken broth to boil.
3. Remove saucepan from heat and add the couscous, stirring constantly with a fork until mixture is thick.
4. Grease a round 2 qt casserole and spoon the couscous into it; using a large spoon push and flatten the couscous up the sides to within 1/2 inch of the rim. Set aside
5. Bring the tomatoes to a simmer in a medium saucepan and add all other ingredients. Cover and simmer for 5 minutes.
6. Spoon the vegetables into the casserole, cover and bake for 1 hour.

Nutritional Information per Serving

Calories	181	Carbohydrates	35 gm
Protein	7 gm	Fat	1 gm
Fiber	9 gm		

Vitamins & Minerals

Iron	3 mg	Vitamin A	1460 RE
Calcium	133 mg	Vitamin C	123 mg

Bean Salad

Serves: 8

1 (15 oz.) can green beans
1 (15 oz.) can yellow wax beans
1 (15 oz.) can garbanzo beans
1 cup onions, chopped
1 cup parsley, chopped
2 tbs oil, Puritan Canola ®
1 (15 oz.) can kidney beans
1 cup green pepper, chopped
1/2 cup pimento, chopped
1 cup celery, chopped
1 cup red wine vinegar

Instructions

1. Pour all beans in a colander and drain well.
2. In a large bowl, combine all vegetables.
3. Bring vinegars and oil to a boil.
4. Pour vinegar mixture over the vegetables.

This will keep for several weeks in the refrigerator.

Nutritional Information per Serving

Calories	201	Carbohydrates	34 gm
Protein	7 gm	Fat	3 gm
Fiber	8 gm		

Vitamins & Minerals

Iron	3 mg	Vitamin A	131 RE
Calcium	80 mg	Vitamin C	37 mg

Garden Vegetable Barley

Serves: 7

2 tbs vegetable oil
1 cup onions, chopped
1 tbs fresh parsley
1/8 tsp pepper
2 cups mushrooms, chopped
1 cup green peppers, diced
1 cup celery, sliced thinly
1 clove garlic, minced
1/2 tsp dried sage
3 cups cooked barley
1 cup carrots, shredded

Instructions

1. In a large saucepan, saute celery, onion and garlic in oil over medium heat 3 to 4 minutes.
2. Add parsley, sage and pepper; mix well.
3. Cook about 3 minutes or until heated through.
4. In 3 qt. microwaveable bowl, combine oil, celery, onion and garlic. Microwave at HIGH about 1 minute 30 seconds. Add remaining ingredients; mix well.
5. Microwave at HIGH about 4 minutes. Stir before serving.

Nutritional Information per Serving

Calories	146	Carbohydrates	29 gm
Protein	1 gm	Fat	3 gm
Fiber	2 gm		

Vitamins & Minerals

Iron	1mg	Vitamin A	455 RE
Calcium	26 mg	Vitamin C	25 mg

Strawberry Sherbert

Serves: 4

1-1/2 cups frozen strawberries
1 egg white
1-1/4 cups fresh orange juice

Instructions

1. Whirl berries in food processor until smooth.
2. Add orange juice and egg white; mix.
3. Pour into 2 ice cube trays and cover lightly with foil.
4. Place in freezer and freeze until solid.
5. 1 tray at a time, break the cubes into container of food processor and whirl to creamy, smooth texture.
6. Scoop the still soft mixture into 4 serving dishes, cover with foil and freeze up to 1-1/2 hours. Do not let sherbet become frozen solid.

Nutritional Information per Serving

Calories	61	Carbohydrates	13 gm
Protein	2 gm	Fat	1 gm
Fiber	1 gm		

Vitamins & Minerals

Iron	1 mg	Vitamin A	9 RE
Calcium	143 mg	Vitamin C	58 mg

Macaroni Salad

Serves: 4

2 cups cooked macaroni
1-1/2 tbs lemon juice
1 cup celery, diced
1/2 cup carrots, shredded
1/2 cup tomato, diced
3 tbs sour cream, non-fat
1 tbs oil
1/2 cup onions, diced
1/2 cup parsley, minced
1/2 cup green pepper, diced
1/2 tsp black pepper

Instructions

1. Combine oil and lemon juice; beat well
2. Pour over macaroni.
3. Combine onions, celery, parsley, carrots, green pepper and tomato; add pepper and sour cream.
4. Add the vegetable mixture to the macaroni and toss well.
5. Refrigerate for several hours.

Nutritional Information per Serving

Calories	124	Carbohydrates	19 gm
Protein	3 gm	Fat	4 gm
Fiber	2 gm		

Vitamins & Minerals

Iron	2 mg	Vitamin A	477 RE
Calcium	56 mg	Vitamin C	33 mg

Eggplant Lasagna

Serves: 4

2 tbs lemon juice
1 eggplant, medium, unpeeled, halved lengthwise and sliced 1/4 inch thick
2 - 8 oz. cans tomato sauce
1 - 14 -1/2 oz. can tomatoes, chopped
1/3 cup fine dry bread crumbs
1/4 cup mozzarella, part skim milk
1 tbs olive oil
2 garlic cloves, minced
1/4 tsp red pepper flakes
1/4 tsp dried oregano
1/4 tsp dried basil
1/4 cup parmesan cheese
1/2 cup ricotta, part skim

Instructions

1. Preheat broiler
2. In a small bowl, combine lemon juice and olive oil.
3. Brush eggplant slices with the mixture and arrange in a single layer on a nonstick baking sheet.
4. Broil 5 to 6 inches from the heat for 2-1/2 minutes on each side or until golden brown.
5. Reduce the oven temperature to 350 degrees.
6. In a medium bowl, mix the tomato sauce, tomatoes, garlic, red pepper flakes, oregano and basil.
7. In a small bowl, combine the bread crumbs and parmesan cheese.
8. Spoon 1/3 of the tomato sauce into a deep 1-1/2 qt. casserole, sprinkle with 1/3 of the bread crumb mixture, cover with eggplant. Spread 1/2 of the ricotta over the eggplant and continue to layer.
9. Scatter the mozzarella over the top and bake for 45 minutes.

10 Increase the heat to broil and heat for 1 minute or until golden.

Nutritional Information per Serving

Calories	205	Carbohydrates	21 gm
Protein	12 gm	Fat	8 gm
Fiber	6 gm		

Vitamins & Minerals

Iron	2 mg	Vitamin A	56 RE
Calcium	269 mg	Vitamin C	18 mg

Spinach Salad

Serves: 4

6 cups spinach, raw, chopped
1 tomato, raw
6 tbs. salad dressing, no oil
2 cucumbers, raw
2 celery stocks, raw

Instructions

1. Combine all vegetables
2. Cover and refrigerate until ready to serve
3. Toss with dressing

Nutritional Information per Serving

Calories	62	Carbohydrates	19 gm
Protein	2 gm	Fat	1 gm
Fiber	6 gm		

Vitamins & Minerals

Iron	3 mg	Vitamin A	608 RE
Calcium	114 mg	Vitamin C	38 mg

Quick Vegetable Barley Soup

Serves: 4

3/4 lb beef, ground
1 garlic clove, raw
14 1/2 oz tomatoes, whole, canned
1/2 cup celery, raw, chopped
2 cubes beefbouillon flavor cubes
1 tsp. herbs, bay leaf, crumbled
1 cup onions, raw, chopped
5 cup water, municipal
1 cup quick quaker barley
1/2 cup carrots, sliced
1/2 tsp. herbs, basil, ground
2 1/2 cup vegetables, mixed

Instructions

1. In 4-qt. saucepan or dutch oven, brown meat.
2. Add onion and garlic; cook until tender. Drain.
3. Stir in remaining ingredients (except frozen vegetables).
4. Cover; bring to a boil.
5. Reduce heat; simmer 10 minutes, stirring occasionally.
6. Add frozen vegetables; cook about 10 minutes or until vegetables are tender.
7. Additional water may be added if soup becomes too thick.

Nutritional Information per Serving

Calories	314	Carbohydrates	58 gm
Protein	11 gm	Fat	4 gm
Fiber	11 gm		

Vitamins & Minerals

Iron	7 mg	Vitamin A	884 RE
Calcium	177 mg	Vitamin C	25 mg

Melon Salad

Serves: 6

2 cup honeydew melon, raw, cubed
1 cup pears, raw, sliced
1/4 cup jelly, mint
1 cup pineapple, chunks
1 cup grapes, raw, slip skin

Instructions

1. In a salad bowl, combine all ingredients except jelly.
2. Melt jelly until soft; pour over fruit.
3. Toss gently.
4. Cover and chill.

Nutritional Information per Serving

Calories	105	Carbohydrates	25 gm
Protein	12 gm	Fat	1 gm
Fiber	2 gm		

Vitamins & Minerals

Iron	1 mg	Vitamin A	175 RE
Calcium	17 mg	Vitamin C	29 mg

Vegetarian Chili with Rice

Serves: 4

1 tbs. oil, Puritan Canola ®
1 carrot, raw
1 sweet red pepper, raw
2 tsp. spice, chili powder
1 tsp. herbs, bay leaf, crumbled
2 cup tomatoes, canned, low sodium
1/2 cup beans, black, cooked, boiled
3 cups rice, brown, long grain
1 cup onions, raw, chopped
3 garlic cloves, raw
2 cup lentils, cooked, boiled
1 tsp. spice, cumin seed
1/8 tsp. spice, pepper,red
1/2 cup chickpeas, cooked
1/2 cup pinto beans,cooked

Instructions

1. In heavy 6-qt. dutch oven, heat vegetable oil over moderately low heat for 1 minute; add onion, carrot, garlic, and green pepper.
2. Cook, covered, for 10 minutes or until vegetables are soft.
3. Add the lentils, chili powder, cumin, bay leaf, cayenne pepper, and tomatoes, along with a small amount of water if mixture is too thick.
4. Cover and simmer for 10 minutes.
5. Add chickpeas, black beans, and pinto beans; cover and simmer for 30 minutes or until lentils are tender.
6. Before chili is done, cook the rice following package directions, omitting the salt.
7. Ladle the chili over the rice.

Nutritional Information per Serving

Calories	420	Carbohydrates	76 gm
Protein	17gm	Fat	5 gm
Fiber	12 gm		

Vitamins & Minerals

Iron	7 mg	Vitamin A	813 RE
Calcium	107 mg	Vitamin C	59 mg

Mushroom Pilaf Soup

Serves: 10

1 tbs. oil, Puritan Canola ®
1 cup raw onions, chopped, cooked
5 cups water, municipal
2 pkt. bouillon, chicken flavor
2 1/2 cups beans, green, cooked
1/2 tsp. salt, lite
2 carrots, raw
2 garlic cloves, raw
2 cups mushrooms, raw,
1 cup quick quaker barley
2 tbs. vinegar, red wine
1/8 tsp. spice, pepper, black

Instructions

1. In 4-qt. saucepan or dutch oven, saute carrots, onions and garlic in oil over medium heat 3 to 4 minutes or until onions are tender.
2. Add remaining ingredients; mix well.
3. Bring to a boil.
4. Cover; reduce heat.
5. Simmer 18 to 20 minutes or until barley is tender, stirring occasionally.
6. Additional water may be added if soup becomes too thick upon standing.

Nutritional Information per Serving

Calories	94	Carbohydrates	18 gm
Protein	1 gm	Fat	2 gm
Fiber	3 gm		

Vitamins & Minerals

Iron	1 mg	Vitamin A	423 RE
Calcium	31 mg	Vitamin C	6 mg

Whole Wheat Blueberry Waffles

Serves: 4

2 cups milk, skim
1/2 cup egg substitute, frozen
1 cup flour, white
1 cup flour, whole wheat
1/4 tsp. salt, lite, mixture, morton
2 tbs. lemon juice
1 cup blueberries, raw
1 tsp. orange peel, raw
3 tbs. oil, canola, puritan
2 tsp. baking powder

Instructions

1. Heat waffle iron; brush with oil (lightly) if necessary.
2. Beat all ingredients except blueberries, just until smooth.
3. Stir in blueberries.
4. Pour batter from cup onto hot waffle iron.
5. Bake about 5 minutes or until steaming stops.
6. Remove waffle carefully.

Nutritional Information per Serving

Calories	372	Carbohydrates	55 gm
Protein	14gm	Fat	11gm
Fiber	5 gm		

Vitamins & Minerals

Iron	3 mg	Vitamin A	109 RE
Calcium	324 mg	Vitamin C	9 mg

Special Vegetable Salad

Serves: 4

2 cups asparagus, raw, cuts spears
1/4 lb. squash, summer, all varieties
1/2 tsp. herbs, thyme, ground
2 1/2 tsp. oil, canola, puritan
1/4 cup onions, raw, chopped
1/2 cup cauliflower, raw
1 carrot, raw, sliced
1 tbs. shallots, raw, chopped
1/4 tsp. spice, pepper, black
1 1/2 tsp. vinegar, red wine

Instructions

1. Bring 2 quarts unsalted water to a boil; add the asparagus, cauliflower, squash and carrot.
2. Cook for 2 minutes .
3. Drain and rinse under cold water to stop the cooking and drain again.
4. In medium bowl, combine oil, shallots, thyme and pepper.
5. Add the hot vegetables and the onion and toss well.
6. Cover and chill in the refrigerator for 2 to 3 hours, tossing occasionally.
7. Just before serving, stir in the vinegar and toss well.

Nutritional Information per Serving

Calories	119	Carbohydrates	8 gm
Protein	2 gm	Fat	9 gm
Fiber	3 gm		

Vitamins & Minerals

Iron	1 mg	Vitamin A	403 RE
Calcium	45 mg	Vitamin C	30 mg

Banana Bread

Serves: 4

1/2 cup margarine, extra light,sunflower	1 cup sugar, white
1/4 cup egg substitute, frozen	2 cups flour, white
1/4 cup walnuts, dried, chips	1 tsp. baking soda
3 bananas, raw	

Instructions

1.Cream margarine, sugar and eggs.
2. Add flour, soda and walnuts.
3. Crush and beat bananas well; add to batter.
4. Bake in loaf pan, approximately 1 hour at 325 degrees. (May need an additional 15 minutes)

Nutritional Information per Serving

Calories	613	Carbohydrates	108 gm
Protein	9 gm	Fat	16 gm
Fiber	4 gm		

Vitamins & Minerals

Iron	3 mg	Vitamin A	223 RE
Calcium	117 mg	Vitamin C	8 mg

Fruit Salad

Serves: 4

2 bananas, raw
1 cup strawberries, raw
1 1/2 tbs. juice, calcium fortified orange
2 oranges, raw, Florida
8 tbs. sour cream, non-fat
1 cup cereal, Health Valley ®

Instructions

1. Mix sour cream, sweetener and orange juice.
2. Arrange fruit in 4 dishes.
3. Top with sour cream mixture and sprinkle with cereal.

Nutritional Information per Serving

Calories	176	Carbohydrates	35 gm
Protein	4 gm	Fat	2 gm
Fiber	5 gm		

Vitamins & Minerals

Iron	1 mg	Vitamin A	61 RE
Calcium	105 mg	Vitamin C	63 mg

Boiled Shrimp

Serves: 4

2 lb. shrimp, raw
1/4 cup onions, raw, chopped
1 tsp. herbs, bay leaf, crumbled
1/8 tsp. red cayenne pepper
1/2 lemon, raw, without peel
8 cups water, municipal
1 garlic clove, raw
1/4 cup celery, raw, diced
1 tsp. salt

Instructions

1. Devein, wash and drain shrimp.
2. Add shrimp to water with the seasoning.
3. Slice and add the 1/2 lemon.
4. Simmer shrimp for 15 minutes.
5. Cool in water.
6. Drain and chill.

Nutritional Information per Serving

Calories	252	Carbohydrates	4 gm
Protein	49 gm	Fat	5 gm
Fiber	T		

Vitamins & Minerals

Iron	5 mg	Vitamin A	129 RE
Calcium	145 mg	Vitamin C	6 mg

Lemon Catfish in Foil

Serves: 4

1 lb. catfish, raw
1/ 3 cup lemon juice, raw
1/2 cup carrots, frozen, sliced
1/4 cup scallion, raw, tops & bulb
2 lemons, raw, without peel
1 tbs. margarine, extra light
1/2 tsp. spice, pepper, black
1/4 cup celery,raw, diced
2 tsp. herbs, parsley, dried

Instructions

1. Place catfish on a piece of foil that is about 4" longer than the fish.
2. Melt margarine and add lemon juice, pepper, carrots, celery, onions, and parsley.
3. Pour the mixture over the fish dividing it evenly.
4. Top the fish with the lemon slices.
5. Bring the edges of foil together and fold over several times.
6. Twist one end of the foil to make it look like a fish tail.
7. Tuck the other end under to form a point to make it look like the nose of the catfish.
8. Place on a cookie sheet and bake at 350 degrees for about 30 minutes or until fish flakes easily.

Nutritional Information per Serving

Calories	173	Carbohydrates	5 gm
Protein	23 gm	Fat	7 gm
Fiber	1 gm		

Vitamins & Minerals

Iron	2 mg	Vitamin A	440 RE
Calcium	69 mg	Vitamin C	32 mg

Pita Pizza

Serves: 1

1 pita bread, jumbo whole wheat
2 oz. cheese, mozzarella, part skim
1/4 cup onions, raw, chopped
1/2 cup tomato sauce
1/4 cup mushrooms, raw

Instructions

1. Slice open pita bread and lay on oven cooking pan.
2. Spread tomato sauce, cheese, mushrooms and onions over the two halves.
3. Place oven on broil.
4. Broil pita halves until light brown.

Nutritional Information per Serving

Calories	424	Carbohydrates	58 gm
Protein	27 gm	Fat	9 gm
Fiber	14 gm		

Vitamins & Minerals

Iron	3 mg	Vitamin A	101 RE
Calcium	527 mg	Vitamin C	17 mg

Stuffed Squash

Serves: 4

8 summer squash, cooked, boiled
2 1/2 cups rice, brown, long grain
1 tsp. spice, cinnamon, ground
1 tsp. spice, pepper, black
1 cup tofu, regular
1/3 cup tomato sauce, no salt
1 tsp. spice, garlic powder
1 qt. tomato puree, no salt

Instructions

1. Clean out the inside of eight summer squash.
2. Fill the insides with the following :
   - 1 package of tofu crumbles
   - 2 1/2 cups of cooked brown rice
3. Sprinkle with cinnamon, pepper, and garlic salt.
4. Add 1/3 cup of tomato sauce.
5. Mix all ingredients and stuff squash.
6. Put the squash in a pan and pour a 29 oz can of tomato puree over the squash.
7. Bring to a boil and simmer on low for 45 minutes.

Nutritional Information per Serving

Calories	307	Carbohydrates	56 gm
Protein	11 gm	Fat	3 gm
Fiber	11 gm		

Vitamins & Minerals

Iron	8 mg	Vitamin A	322 RE
Calcium	166 mg	Vitamin C	98 mg

Hummus Tahini

Serves: 4

15 oz. beans, dried, chickpeas
1 garlic clove, raw
4 pieces of pita bread, whole wheat
2 tbs. sesame butter, paste
3 tbs. lemon juice, raw

Instructions

1. Put puree beans in blender with 4 tbs. of water.
2. Add the juice of one lemon, and one clove of garlic crushed.
3. Add two tbs. tahini.
4. Mix all ingredients in blender.
5. Spread mixture over pita bread.

Nutritional Information per Serving

Calories	318	Carbohydrates	58 gm
Protein	11 gm	Fat	5 gm
Fiber	9 gm		

Vitamins & Minerals

Iron	4 mg	Vitamin A	3 RE
Calcium	154 mg	Vitamin C	9 mg

Cheese Tomato & Lettuce Sandwich

Serves:1

2 slices bread, oat, country
3 slices tomatoes, raw
1 tsp. spicy, yellow mustard
1 slice cheese, Lite-Line ®
1 lettuce leaf, raw

Instructions

1. Toast sliced bread.
2. Spread mustard over toasted bread.
3. Add cheese, tomatoes, and lettuce.

Nutritional Information per Serving

Calories	236	Carbohydrates	32 gm
Protein	14 gm	Fat	6 gm
Fiber	4 gm		

Vitamins & Minerals

Iron	2 mg	Vitamin A	59 RE
Calcium	197 mg	Vitamin C	9 mg

Lentils and Rice

Serves: 4

3 cups lentils, cooked, boiled
1 cup onions, raw, chopped
1 tbs. olive oil
4 cups rice, brown, cooked
1 garlic clove, raw

Instructions

1. Combine rice, lentils and crushed clove of garlic.
2. Put into covered pot with lid.
3. Fill with water until ingredients are covered.
4. Bring to a boil.
5. Cook on low for 45 minutes.
6. In another sauce pan, saute onions in the olive oil until soft.
7. Add onions to cooked lentils and rice.
8. If desired, add salt and pepper for taste.

Nutritional Information per Serving

Calories	447	Carbohydrates	84 gm
Protein	17 gm	Fat	5 gm
Fiber	8 gm		

Vitamins & Minerals

Iron	6 mg	Vitamin A	2 RE
Calcium	63 mg	Vitamin C	6 mg

Asparagus and Shrimp Salad

Serves: 4

1 1/2 lbs. asparagus, raw, cooked
4 tbs. mayonnaise, low-fat
1/2 tsp. lemon juice, canned or bottled
1/2 tsp. horseradish, prepared
12 lettuce leaves, raw
5 pieces shrimp
4 tbs. sour cream, non-fat
1/4 tsp. spice, mustard seed
1/2 tsp. spice, pepper,black
1/2 tbs. water

Instructions

1. Blanche asparagus, drain on paper towels.
2. Cut off tips; cut stems diagonally into 2 inch pieces.
3. Place tips and stems with shrimp in a large bowl.
4. Combine mayonnaise with sour cream in a medium bowl.
5. Beat in lemon juice, horseradish, mustard, water, salt and pepper to taste.
6. Spoon dressing over asparagus and shrimp, toss well.
7. Serve on lettuce leaves at room temperature or slightly chilled.

Nutritional Information per Serving

Calories	110	Carbohydrates	10 gm
Protein	6 gm	Fat	5 gm
Fiber	4 gm		

Vitamins & Minerals

Iron	2 mg	Vitamin A	187 RE
Calcium	83 mg	Vitamin C	37 mg

Eggplant and Tomato Casserole

Serves: 4

1 eggplant, cooked, boiled, drained
2/3 cup onions, raw, chopped
1 tbs. cheese, parmesan, grated
1 pepper, green, raw,
2 cups tomatoes, raw
1 tsp. seasoning, blend

Instructions

1. Peel and dice eggplant.
2. Parboil for 5 minutes and drain well.
3. Place eggplant, pepper, onion, tomatoes, parmesan cheese and seasoning into a lightly oiled casserole.
4. Bake at 350 degrees for 35 to 40 minutes.

Nutritional Information per Serving

Calories	76	Carbohydrates	15 gm
Protein	2 gm	Fat	1 gm
Fiber	5 gm		

Vitamins & Minerals

Iron	2 mg	Vitamin A	123 RE
Calcium	39 mg	Vitamin C	45 mg

Skillet Dinner

Serves: 8

2 tbs. oil, Puritan Canola ®
1 pepper, green, raw, sweet
2 tbs. spice, chili powder
2 cups kidney beans, red, dried
4 cups tomatoes, canned, whole
2 oz. cheese, monterey jack
3/4 cup onions, raw, chopped
2 garlic cloves, raw
1/2 tsp. spice, cumin seed
10 oz. yellow corn,cut off cob
4 cups pasta, macaroni

Instructions

1. In large skillet, heat oil over medium- high heat.
2. Add onion, green pepper, garlic, chili powder and cumin; cook 4 minutes or until vegetables are tender.
3. Add kidney beans, corn and tomatoes with juice.
4. Bring to a boil.
5. Reduce heat and simmer, stirring occasionally, for 15 minutes.
6. Toss with macaroni; sprinkle with cheese.

Nutritional Information per Serving

Calories	279	Carbohydrates	44 gm
Protein	11gm	Fat	6 gm
Fiber	10 gm		

Vitamins & Minerals

Iron	4.5 mg	Vitamin A	175 RE
Calcium	123 mg	Vitamin C	35 mg

Garden Pie

Serves: 6

2 cups squash, summer, raw	1 cup tomatoes, raw, diced
2 oz. cheese, swiss	1/3 cup onions, raw, chopped
2 cups skim milk	1/4 cup egg substitute, frozen
1 cup baking mix, bisquick	1/3 cup cheese, parmesan
1/4 tsp. salt, lite salt, mixture	1/10 tsp. spice, pepper, black

Instructions

1. Grease a 10x1-1/2 " pie plate
2. Sprinkle zucchini, tomato, swiss cheese and onion in plate.
3. Beat remaining ingredients 15 seconds in blender on high for one minute with hand beater or until smooth.
4. Pour into plate.
5. Bake 35 to 40 minutes, or until knife inserted in center comes out clean.
6. Cool 5 minutes.
7. Garnish with tomato and zucchini slices, if desired.

Nutritional Information per Serving

Calories	186	Carbohydrates	22 gm
Protein	11 gm	Fat	6 gm
Fiber	2 gm		

Vitamins & Minerals

Iron	1.4 mg	Vitamin A	147 RE
Calcium	289 mg	Vitamin C	11 mg

Vegetable and Rice Casserole

Serves: 4

1 tbs. olive oil
1 garlic clove, raw
1 pepper, sweet, raw, red
1/2 tsp. spice, paprika
2 1/2 cups rice, white, w/out salt & fat
1/2 lb. squash, summer, zucchini
2 cups peas, green, raw, cooked
3/4 cup onions, raw, chopped
1 tomato, raw
1 potato, w/out skin, boiled
1/4 tsp. spice, pepper, red
2 cups soup, chicken broth
2 carrots, raw

Instructions

1. In large saucepan, heat olive oil over moderate heat for 1 minute.
2. Add the onion and garlic; cook, stirring, for 1 minute.
3. Mix in the tomato and pepper and cook for 3 minutes.
4. Add the potato, paprika, and cayenne pepper and cook for 2 minutes.
5. Stir in rice and chicken broth and bring to a boil; simmer gently.
6. Cover and simmer for 15 minutes, or until most liquid is absorbed.
7. Stir in zucchini, carrots, and peas; cover and cook for 10 minutes.

Nutritional Information per Serving

Calories	301	Carbohydrates	56 gm
Protein	8 gm	Fat	5 gm
Fiber	7 gm		

Vitamins & Minerals

Iron	3 mg	Vitamin A	1241 RE
Calcium	59 mg	Vitamin C	66 mg

Broccoli Supreme

Serves: 6

3 cups broccoli, chopped
3 cups rice, white, w/out salt
3/4 cup celery, raw, diced pieces
3/4 cup peppers, sweet, red, raw
2 oz. cheese, lite-line
4 tbs. margarine, extra light
3/4 cup onions, raw, chopped
2 cups soup, cream of mush.

Instructions

1. Cook rice.
2. Add cheese and mix well.
3. Saute celery, green pepper, and onion in margarine.
4. Add broccoli and soup; mix thoroughly.
5. Pour into greased 9 x 13" baking dish.
6. Bake at 350 degrees for 1 hour.

Nutritional Information per Serving

Calories	263	Carbohydrates	33 gm
Protein	8 gm	Fat	11 gm
Fiber	5 gm		

Vitamins & Minerals

Iron	2 mg	Vitamin A	314 RE
Calcium	149 mg	Vitamin C	64 mg

Squash Casserole

Serves: 6

6 cups squash, summer, all varieties
1 1/2 cups carrots, raw, sliced
1 cup soup, cream of mushroom
4 oz. cheese, cheddar, sharp
2 tbs. margarine, extra light
1 1/2 cups onions, raw
1 1/2 cups peppers, red, raw
8 oz. sour cream, non-fat
4 oz. stuffing, herb seasoned
1/4 tsp. spice, pepper, black

Instructions

1. Mix crumbs with margarine; sprinkle 1/2 crumbs on bottom of casserole dish.
2. Cook squash, onion, carrot and pepper until done; drain.
3. Add pepper; mash slightly.
4. Add soup, sour cream and cheese; mix thoroughly.
5. Pour mixture into casserole.
6. Sprinkle remaining crumbs on top.
7. Bake at 375 degrees for 25 - 30 minutes.

Nutritional Information per Serving

Calories	219	Carbohydrates	24 gm
Protein	10gm	Fat	9 gm
Fiber	5 gm		

Vitamins & Minerals

Iron	1.4 mg	Vitamin A	1261 RE
Calcium	314 mg	Vitamin C	52 mg

FOOD VALUE

TABLES

(Most of the food values were provided by the U.S. Department of Agriculture)

DESCRIPTION	SERV SIZE	KCAL	FAT (gm)	PROT (gm)	CARB (gm)	FIBER (gm)	VIT-A (RE)	VIT-C (mg)
BEVERAGES								
Beer	12 oz.	146	0	.9	13.2	.70	0	0
Wine	3.5 oz	70	0	.1	.8	0	0	0
Cola beverage	12 oz.	151	0	.1	38.5	0	0	0
Diet Cola	12 oz.	2	0	.2	.3	0	0	0
Coffee, instant	1 cup	2.5	0	.3	.9	0	0	0
Fruit punch, can	1 cup	118	.06	.1	30.1	0	4	75
Lemonade, frozen	1 cup	100	.10	.1	26	.29	5	10
Tea, brewed	1 cup	2.5	0	.1	.5	0	0	0
Tea, instant	1 cup	2.5	0	.1	.4	0	0	0
DAIRY								
Cheddar cheese	1 oz.	114	9.4	7.1	.4	0	86	0
Cottage, small curd	1 cup	215	8.93	26	5.6	0	101	0
Mozzarella:								
with whole milk	1 oz.	80	5.76	5.5	.6	0	68	0
with skim milk	1 oz.	80	4.68	7.6	.9	0	54	0
Ricotta, whole milk	1 cup	428	31.9	27.7	7.5	0	330	0
American cheese	1 oz.	106	8.8	6.3	.5	0	82	0
Swiss cheese	1 oz.	95	6.98	7	.6	0	62	0
Cream:								
Half & Half	1 tbsp.	20	1.7	.4	.7	0	16	0
whipping	1 tbsp.	44	4.6	.3	.4	0	44	0
Sour cream	1 tbsp.	30	2.93	.4	.6	0	27	0
Sour cream, imit.	1 tbsp.	29	2.73	.3	.9	0	0	0
Milk, whole	1 cup	150	8.15	8	11	0	76	2
Milk, 2%	1 cup	121	4.78	8.1	11.7	0	140	2
Milk, 1%	1 cup	102	2.54	8	11.7	0	145	2
Milk, skim	1 cup	86	.44	8.3	11.9	0	149	2
Buttermilk	1 cup	99	2.16	8.1	11.7	0	20	2
Milk shake, choc.	10 oz.	360	10.5	9.6	57.9	.29	64	1
Milk deserts:								
Ice cream	1 cup	269	14.3	4.8	31.7	0	133	1
Ice milk	1 cup	184	5.6	5.2	29	0	52	1
Soft serve	1 cup	223	4.6	8	38.4	0	44	1
Sherbert	1 cup	270	3.8	2.2	58.7	0	39	4
Custard	1 cup	305	15	14	29	0	146	1
Yogurt, lowfat	1 cup	144	3.5	11.9	16	0	36	2
EGGS								
Fried in butter	1 ea.	95	6.4	5.4	.5	0	94	0
Hardboiled	1 ea.	79	5.6	6.1	.6	0	78	0
Poached	1 ea.	79	5.5	6	.6	0	78	0

DESCRIPTION	SERV SIZE	KCAL	FAT (gm)	PROT (gm)	CARB (gm)	FIBER (gm)	VIT-A (RE)	VIT-C (mg)
FATS and OILS								
Butter	1 tbsp.	100	11.5	.1	0	0	106	0
Margarine:								
soft (80%)	1 tbsp.	100	11.4	1.1	0	0	140	0
hard (80%)	1 tbsp.	100	11.4	.1	.1	0	139	0
imitation (40%)	1 tbsp.	50	5.5	0	0	0	141	0
Oils:								
corn	1 tbsp.	125	14	0	0	0	0	0
olive	1 tbsp.	125	14	0	0	0	0	0
peanut	1 tbsp.	125	14	0	0	0	0	0
sunflower	1 tbsp.	125	14	0	0	0	0	0
Salad dressings:								
blue cheese	1 tbsp.	75	8	.7	1.1	.01	10	0
french, reg.	1 tbsp.	85	9	0	1	.13	0	0
french, low cal	1 tbsp.	75	2	0	2.5	.05	0	0
italian, reg.	1 tbsp.	80	9	.1	1	.03	0	0
italian, low cal	1 tbsp.	5	.5	0	.7	.04	0	0
thousand island	1 tbsp.	60	5.7	.1	2.4	.03	15	0
Mayonnaise:								
regular	1 tbsp.	100	11	.2	.4	0	12	0
imitation	1 tbsp.	35	3	0	2	0	0	0
Tartar sauce	1 tbsp.	74	8.1	.2	.6	.04	9	0
FRUITS								
Apple, 3 1/4" diam.	1 ea.	125	.8	.4	32	6.58	11	12
Apple juice	1 cup	116	.3	.1	29	.52	0	2
Apple sauce, juice	1 cup	106	.1	.4	27	5.12	7	3
Apricots, raw	3 ea.	51	.4	1.5	11.8	2.23	277	10.6
Apricot nectar	1 cup	141	.2	.9	36.1	1.51	330	2
Avocado, mashed	1 cup	370	35.2	4.6	17	6.43	141	18
Banana, 8 inch	1 ea.	105	.5	1.2	26.7	3.26	9	10
Blackberries, raw	1 cup	74	.6	1	18.4	9.72	24	30
Blueberries, raw	1 cup	82	.6	1	20.5	4.93	15	20
Dates, whole	10 ea..	228	.4	1.6	61	7.2	9	0
Figs, dried	10 ea.	477	2.2	5.7	122	24	25	1
Fruit cocktail:								
heavy syrup	1 cup	185	.2	1	48.2	2.52	52	5
juice pack	1 cup	115	0	1.1	29.4	2.52	76	7
Grapefruit, 3-3/4 in:								
Pink	1 half	37	.1	.7	9.4	1.53	32	47
white	1 half	39	.1	.8	9.9	1.46	1	39
Grapefruit juice:								
raw	1 cup	96	.2	1.2	22.7	.37	2	94
can, unsweet	1 cup	93	.2	1.3	22.1	.25	2	72
can, sweetened	1 cup	115	.2	1.4	27.8	.25	2	67

DESCRIPTION	SERV SIZE	KCAL	FAT (gm)	PROT (gm)	CARB (gm)	FIBER (gm)	VIT-A (RE)	VIT-C (mg)
FRUITS								
Grapes:								
Thompson	10 ea.	35	.3	.3	8.9	1	4	5
Tokay/Emperor	10 ea.	40	.3	.4	10.1	1	4	6
Grape juice:								
Bottled or can	1 cup	155	.2	1.4	37.9	1.26	2	0
Kiwi fruit	1 ea.	46	.3	.8	11.3	1.16	13	74
Lemon, raw	1 ea.	17	.2	.6	5.4	1.19	2	31
Mango, raw	1 ea.	135	.6	1.1	35.2	2.86	806	57
Cantalope, 5 in.	1 half	94	.7	2.4	22.3	2.67	861	113
Nectarines, raw	1 ea.	67	.6	1.3	11.8	1.40	5	32
Oranges, raw	1 ea.	60	.2	1.2	15.4	2.97	27	70
Orange, juice	1 cup	111	.5	1.7	25.8	.5	50	124
Papaya, raw	1 cup	60	.2	.9	13.7	2.38	282	92
Peaches, raw	1 ea.	37	0	.6	9.6	2	47	6
Peach, w/syrup	1 cup	190	.2	1.2	51	4.2	85	7
Pears, raw	1 ea.	98	.7	.7	25.1	4.98	3	7
Pears, w/syrup	1 cup	188	.3	.5	48.9	5	1	3
Pineapple, raw	1 cup	76	.7	.6	19.2	2.95	4	24
Pineapple, w/syrup	1 cup	199	.3	.9	51.5	2.43	4	19
Plums, raw, med.	1 ea.	36	.4	.5	8.6	1.4	21	6
Plums, w/syrup	1 cup	230	.3	.9	60	4.4	67	1
Prunes, raw	10 ea.	201	.4	2.2	52.7	13.5	167	3
Prune juice	1 cup	181	0	1.6	44.7	3	0	11
Raisins, seedless	1 cup	435	.7	4.7	115	9.6	1	5
Raspberries, raw	1 cup	60	.7	1.1	14.2	9.1	16	31
Rhubarb, w/sugar	1 cup	279	.1	.9	74.9	5.28	17	8
Strawberries, raw	1 cup	45	.6	.9	10.5	3.28	4	85
Tangerines, raw	1 ea.	37	.2	.5	9.4	1.6	77	26
Watermelon, diced	1 cup	50	.7	1	11.5	.80	59	15
BREADS, ROLLS, COOKIES and DESSERTS								
Bagel, 3 1/4 in.	1 ea.	200	1.75	7.5	38.2	.74	0	0
Bisquit, from mix	1 ea.	94	3.1	2.1	13.7	.6	4	0
Breads:								
Boston brown	1 pce.	95	.62	2	21	1.7	0	0
Cracked wheat	1 pce.	65	.87	2.3	12.5	1.2	0	0
French, 5x2x1	1 pce	100	1.36	3.3	17.7	.58	0	0
Oatmeal bread	1 pce.	65	1.1	2.1	12	.86	0	0
Pita, pocket	1 ea.	165	.88	6.2	33	.69	0	0
Pumpernickel	1 pce.	80	1.1	2.9	15.4	1.33	0	0
Raisin	1 pce.	68	1	1.9	13.2	.68	0	0
Rye	1 pce.	65	.9	2.1	12	1.6	0	0
Wheat	1 pce.	65	1	2.4	11.8	1.4	0	0
White	1 pce.	65	1	2.1	12.2	.68	0	0

DESCRIPTION	SERV SIZE	KCAL	FAT (gm)	PROT (gm)	CARB (gm)	FIBER (gm)	VIT-A (RE)	VIT-C (mg)
BREADS, ROLLS, COOKIES and DESSERTS, cont'd.								
Bread, cont'd.								
Whole wheat	1 pce.	70	1.2	3	12.7	3.17	0	0
Cakes:								
Angel food	1 pce.	125	.2	3.2	28.5	.25	0	0
Coffee	1 pce.	230	6.9	4.5	37.7	.54	32	0
Devil's food	1 pce.	235	8	3	40.2	.32	31	0
Gingerbread	1 pce.	174	4.3	2	32.2	.34	0	0
Fruitcake	1 pce.	165	7.	2	25	1.2	13	16
Pound cake	1 pce.	110	5.4	2	15	.22	41	0
Cookies:								
Brownies	1 ea.	95	6.3	1.3	11	.20	6	0
Choc. chip	4 ea.	180	8.8	2.3	28	.17	15	0
Fig bars	4 ea.	210	3.8	2	42.3	.80	6	0
Corn chips	1 oz.	155	9	2	16	.3	11	1
Crackers:								
Graham	2 ea.	60	1.5	1	10.8	1.4	0	0
Saltines	4 ea.	50	1.1	1	9	.06	0	0
wheat	4 ea.	35	1.4	1	5	.4	0	0
Croissant	1 ea.	235	12	5	27	.47	13	0
Danish:								
Round w/fruit	1 ea.	235	13	4	28	.65	11	0
Doughnut, plain	1 ea.	210	12	2.5	24	.5	5	0
English muffin	1 ea.	140	1.1	4.5	26.2	1.5	0	0
Muffins, mix:								
Blueberry	1 ea.	140	4.9	2.7	22	1.2	11	.5
Bran	1 ea.	140	4	3	24	2.0	14	0
Cornmeal	1 ea.	145	6	3	22	1.6	16	0
Pancakes:								
Buckwheat	1 ea.	55	2	2	6	1.3	17	0
plain	1 ea.	60	2	2	8	.72	7	0
Pie crust, 9 in.	shell	900	60	11	79	3.6	0	0
Pies, 9 in.:								
Apple	1 pce.	405	17.5	3.7	59.5	3.13	30	0
Banana cream	1 pce.	320	12.9	6.3	47.2	1.7	37	3
Cherry	1 pce.	410	17.8	4.3	60.5	2.4	114	1
Choc. cream	1 pce.	311	12.7	7	42.5	.73	34	.5
Custard	1 pce.	293	14.2	7	34	.6	64	0
Lemon meringue	1 pce.	355	14.3	4.7	53	.76	73	4
Peach	1 pce.	405	17.5	3.5	60.7	2.83	93	5
Pecan	1 pce.	583	23.7	6.3	91.8	1.6	41.7	0
Pumpkin	1 pce.	375	15.7	9	51.3	2.5	1861	1
Pretzels:								
Thin sticks	10 ea.	10	.1	.3	2.4	.07	0	0
Dutch twists	1 ea.	65	.6	1.5	12.8	.36	0	0

DESCRIPTION	SERV SIZE	KCAL	FAT (gm)	PROT (gm)	CARB (gm)	FIBER (gm)	VIT-A (RE)	VIT-C (mg)
BREADS, ROLLS, COOKIES and DESSERTS, cont'd.								
Rolls & Buns:								
Hotdog bun	1 ea.	115	2.1	3.3	20	1.08	0	0
Hamburger bun	1 ea.	129	2.4	3.7	22.5	1.2	0	0
Submarine roll	1 ea.	400	8	11	72	2.2	0	0
Dinner roll	1 ea.	120	3	3	20	.9	8	0
Tortillas:								
Corn, 6 in.	1 ea.	65	1	2	13	1.2	8	0
Flour, 8 in.	1 ea.	105	2.7	2.6	19	.9	0	0
Taco shell	1 ea.	48	2.2	.9	7	.7	4	0
Waffles	1 ea.	205	8	7	27	1.6	49	0
GRAINS								
Barley, cooked	1 cup	196	.6	4.6	44	4.4	0	0
Breakfast, hot:								
Yellow grits	1 cup	146	.5	3.5	31.4	.7	15	0
White, instant	1 cup	80	.2	2	17.8	.4	0	0
Cream of Wheat	1 cup	140	.6	3.6	29	.6	0	0
Oatmeal	1 cup	145	2	6	25	9.2	4	0
Breakfast, cold:								
All-Bran ®	1/3 c	70	.5	4	21	8.4	375	15
Cap'n Crunch ®	1 cup	156	3.4	1.9	30	.9	5	0
Cherrio's ®	1 cup	89	1.4	3.4	15.7	.9	304	12
Corn Flakes:								
Kellogg's ®	1 1/4 c	110	0	2.3	24	.5	375	15
40% Bran Flakes:								
Kellogg's ®	1 cup	125	.7	5	30	5	522	0
Fruit Loops ®	1 cup	111	1	1.7	25	.3	375	15
Grape Nuts ®	1/2 cup	202	.2	6.6	26.4	3.31	753	0
Product 19 ®	1 cup	126	.2	3.2	27	.4	500	0
Raisin Bran:								
Kellogg's ®	1 cup	211	1.8	5.3	52.7	5.8	500	0
Post ®	1 cup	174	1	5.3	42.9	6	750	0
Rice Krispies:								
Kellogg's ®	1 cup	112	.2	2	24.8	.12	388	15
Shredd wheat	3/4 cup	115	.8	3.5	25	3.9	0	0
Special K ®	1 1/2 c	125	.1	6	24	.35	429	17
Wheaties ®	1 cup	101	.5	2.8	23.1	3.3	388	15
Macaroni:								
Firm stage, hot	1 cup	190	.7	6.5	39.1	1.04	0	0
Tender, cold	1 cup	115	.4	3.8	24	.84	0	0
Tender, hot	1 cup	155	.7	5	32	1.12	0	0
Noodles:								
Egg noodles	1 cup	200	2	6.6	37	.2	34	0
Chow Mein, dry	1 cup	220	11	6	26	.05	0	0

DESCRIPTION	SERV SIZE	KCAL	FAT (gm)	PROT (gm)	CARB (gm)	FIBER (gm)	VIT-A (RE)	VIT-C (mg)
GRAINS, cont'd.								
Popcorn:								
Air popped, plain	1 cup	30	.4	1	6	1.5	1	0
Popped in oil	1 cup	55	3	.9	6	1.5	2	0
Rice, cooked:								
Brown	1 cup	232	1.2	5	50	4	0	0
White, enriched	1 cup	223	.2	4	50	.8	0	0
Wild	1 cup	184	.4	6	38	5	0	0
Rye Flour	1 cup	392	2	13	85	8	0	0
Spaghetti, cooked:								
Firm stage, hot	1 cup	190	.7	6	39	1.4	0	0
Tender stage,	1 cup	155	.6	5	32	1	0	0
Whole wheat	1 cup	151	.5	7	32	4	0	0
Wheat Flour:								
All purpose, wh.	1 cup	455	1	13	95	3.5	0	0
Cake	1 cup	349	.9	7	76	2.5	0	0
Whole wheat	1 cup	400	2.4	16	85	15.2	0	0
FISH								
Clams, raw meat	3 oz.	65	1	11	.2	.01	26	9
Cod:								
Baked, w/butter	3 oz.	114	6	23	0	0	30	0
Batter fried	3 oz.	199	10	19	7.5	0	0	0
Poached	3 oz.	94	1	21	0	0	0	0
Fish sticks	2 ea.	140	6	12	8	.02	10	0
Haddock, breaded	3 oz.	175	9	17	7	.03	20	0
Oysters, raw	1 cup	160	4	20	8	0	223	24
Salmon:								
Broiled or bake	3 oz.	140	5	21	0	0	87	0
Scallops, breaded	6 ea.	195	10	15	10	.02	21	0
Shrimp:								
Boiled	3 oz.	109	1.5	23	0	0	18	0
Fried	3 oz.	200	10	16	11	.09	26	0
Tuna, canned:								
Oil pack, drain	3 oz.	165	7	24	0	0	20	0
Water packed	3 oz.	135	1	30	0	0	32	0
BEEF, PORK and LAMB								
Beef, cooked:								
Chuck	3 oz.	325	26	22	0	0	.06	0
Round	3 oz.	220	13	25	0	0	0	0
Sirloin	3 oz.	240	15	23	0	0	0	0
Grd. beef	3 oz.	230	16	21	0	0	0	0
Liver, fried	3 oz.	185	7	23	7	0	9120	23

DESCRIPTION	SERV SIZE	KCAL	FAT (gm)	PROT (gm)	CARB (gm)	FIBER (gm)	VIT-A (RE)	VIT-C (mg)
BEEF, PORK and LAMB, cont'd.								
Lamb, cooked:								
Loin chop, bro.	2.8 oz.	235	16	22	0	0	0	0
Leg, roasted	3 oz.	205	13	22	0	0	0	0
Rib, roasted	3 oz.	315	26	18	0	0	0	0
Bacon	3 pce.	109	9.3	5.8	.1	0	0	6
Canadian bacon	2 pce.	86	3.9	11.3	.6	0	0	10
Ham, roasted	3 oz.	207	14.2	18.3	0	0	0	0
Pork, fresh, cooked:								
Chops, broiled	3.1 oz.	275	19.2	23.9	0	0	3	.3
Chops, fried	1 ea.	334	27.2	20.7	0	0	3	.3
Pork leg, roasted	3 oz.	250	18	21	0	0	2	.3
Veal :								
Cutlet, broiled	3 oz.	185	9.4	23	0	0	0	0
Liver, simmered	3 oz.	222	11.2	25.1	3.4	0	6464	31
CHICKEN and TURKEY								
Chicken, cooked:								
Fried, batter dipped:								
Breast, w/bone	5 oz.	364	18.5	34.8	12.6	.05	28	0
Thigh	1 ea.	238	14.2	18.6	7.8	.03	25	0
Fried, flour coated:								
Breast, w/bone	4.2 oz	218	8.7	31.2	1.6	.01	15	0
Thigh	1 ea.	162	9.3	16.6	2	.01	18	0
Roasted:								
Dark meat	1 cup	286	13.6	38.3	0	0	30	0
Light meat	1 cup	242	6.3	43.3	0	0	12	0
Chicken hot dog	1 ea.	115	8.8	5.8	3.1	0	17	0
Turkey patty, fried	1 ea.	181	11.5	9	10	.03	7	0
BOLOGNA, SAUSAGES and LUNCHMEATS								
Bologna:								
Beef and pork	1 pce.	89	8	3.3	.8	0	0	6
Turkey	2 pce.	113	8.6	7.8	.6	0	0	0
Sausage links:								
Brown & serve	1 ea.	50	5	2	.1	0	0	0
Pork links	1 ea.	50	4	2.5	.1	0	0	0
Frankfurter:								
Beef and pork	1 ea.	145	13.1	5.1	1.1	0	0	12
Chicken	1 ea.	115	8.8	5.8	3.1	0	17	0
Turkey	1 ea.	102	8.3	6.4	.7	0	17	0
Ham:								
Lunchmeat	2 pce.	103	6	10	1.8	0	0	16
Turkey ham	2 pce.	75	3	11	.2	0	0	0

DESCRIPTION	SERV SIZE	KCAL	FAT (gm)	PROT (gm)	CARB (gm)	FIBER (gm)	VIT-A (RE)	VIT-C (mg)
NUTS and SEEDS								
Almonds, raw	1 oz.	167	14.8	5.7	5.8	3	0	1
Almond butter	1 tbsp.	101	9.5	2.4	3.4	1.4	0	0
Cashew, roasted	1 oz.	163	13.2	4.3	9.3	1.7	0	0
Cashew butter	1 tbsp.	94	7.9	2.8	4.4	.9	0	0
Coconut:								
Raw, shredded	1 cup	283	26.8	2.7	12	11	0	3
Dried, shredded	1 cup	515	50	5.4	18	19	0	1
Macadamia nuts	1 oz.	204	21.7	2	3.7	1	3	0
Peanuts:								
Oil roast, salted	1 oz.	165	14	7.6	5	2	0	0
Dried, unsalted	1 oz.	161	14	7	4.6	2.6	0	0
Peanut butter	1 tbsp.	95	8	4.6	2.5	1	0	0
Pistachio, dried	1 oz.	164	13.7	5.9	7	1	7	0
Sesame seeds, dry	1/4 cup	221	20.6	10	3.5	6	0	0
Sesame butter	1 tbsp.	91	8.5	2.7	2.7	2	1	1
Sunflower, dry	1/4 cup	205	17.9	8	6.8	2	2	0
Walnuts, black	1 oz.	172	16	6.9	3.4	2.4	8	0
VEGETABLES and LEGUMES								
Alfafa, sprouted	1 cup	10	.2	1.3	1.2	1	5	3
Articoke, globe	1 ea.	53	.2	2.8	12.4	3.9	17	9
Asparagus, cooked	1/2 cup	22	.3	2.3	4	1.6	75	25
Bamboo, can slices	1 cup	25	.5	2.3	4.2	3.26	1	1
Black beans	1 cup	225	.8	15	41	15.4	1	0
Lima beans, thick	1/2 cup	85	.3	5.2	16	4.6	16	11
Lima beans, thin	1/2 cup	94	.3	6	17.5	4.86	15	5
Green beans	1 cup	44	.4	2.4	10	3.1	83	12
Bean sprouts, raw	1 cup	32	.2	3	6	1.7	2	14
Beats, whole	2 ea.	31	0	1	6.7	2	1	6
Blackeyed peas	1 cup	190	.8	12.8	34.5	10.8	3	0
Broccoli, raw	1 cup	24	.3	2.6	4.6	3	136	8
Brussel sprouts	1 cup	60	.8	6	13	5.6	112	97
Cabbage, raw	1 cup	16	.1	.8	3.8	1.6	9	33
Bok choy, cooked	1 cup	20	.3	2.6	3	3	437	44
Carrots, raw	1 cup	31	.1	.7	7	2	202	7
Carrot juice	3/4 cup	73	.3	1.7	17	2.5	316	11
Cauliflower, raw	1/2 cup	12	0	1	2.5	1.3	0	36
Celery, outer stalk	1 ea.	6	0	.3	1.4	.8	5	3
Collards, cooked	1 cup	20	.2	1.6	3.8	4	322	14
Corn, cob, 5 in.	1 ea.	83	1	2.6	19	3.6	17	5
Cucumber	6 slices	4	0	.2	.8	.4	1	1
Dandelion greens	1 cup	35	.6	2.1	6.7	1.4	1229	19
Eggplant, cooked	1 cup	45	.4	1.3	10.6	6	10	2
Garbanzo beans	1 cup	270	4	15	45	8.6	0	0

DESCRIPTION	SERV SIZE	KCAL	FAT (gm)	PROT (gm)	CARB (gm)	FIBER (gm)	VIT-A (RE)	VIT-C (mg)
VEGETABLES and LEGUMES, cont'd.								
Escarole	1 cup	8	.1	.6	1.7	.75	103	3
Jer. Articoke	1 cup	114	0	3	26	1.9	3	6
Kale, cooked	1 cup	42	.5	3.5	7	3.7	962	53
Lentils, cooked	1 cup	215	1	16	38	10	4	0
Lettuce:								
Iceburg	1 cup	7	.1	.6	1.2	.8	19	2
Romaine	1 cup	9	.1	.9	1.3	.9	146	13
Mushrooms, raw	1/2 cup	9	.1	.7	1.6	.7	0	1
Mustard greens	1 cup	21	.3	3.2	3	3	424	35
Navy bean, cooked	1 cup	225	1.1	15	40	16.5	0	0
Okra, cooked	1/2 cup	34	.3	2	7.5	3	47	11
Onions, raw	1 cup	54	.4	1.9	11.7	2.6	0	13
Parsley, raw	1/2 cup	10	0	.7	2	1.9	156	27
Parsnips, cooked	1 cup	125	1.4	2.1	30	4.4	0	20
Peas:								
Green	1/2 cup	63	.2	4	11	7.6	53	8
Split, cooked	1 cup	230	.6	16	42	10	8	0
Pepper:								
Green	1/2 cup	12	.2	.4	2.6	1.07	261	76
Hot green chili	1 ea.	18	0	.9	4.3	1	35	109
Pinto beans	1 cup	265	.8	15	49	18.9	1	0
Potatoes:								
baked w/skin	1 ea.	220	.2	4.7	51	4.4	0	26
Potato chips	14 chips	148	10	1.8	14.7	.5	0	12
Pumpkin, cooked	1 cup	50	.2	2	11.9	3.7	265	12
Red radishes	10 ea.	7	.2	.3	1.6	.9	0	10
Seaweed, kelp	1 oz.	12	.2	.5	2.7	1.4	3	0
Soybeans, cooked	1 cup	235	10.2	19.8	19.5	4	5	0
Spinach, raw	1 cup	12	.2	1.6	2	2.28	376	16
Squash, cooked:								
Acorn	1 cup	83	.2	1.6	21	5.8	63	16
Butternut	1 cup	83	.2	1.8	21.5	4.9	1435	31
Crookneck	1 cup	36	.6	1.6	7.8	3.2	52	10
Zucchini	1 cup	29	0	1.1	7	3	43	8
Sweet potatoes	1 cup	160	.45	2	37	3.9	2575	26
Tofu	1 pce.	86	5	9	2.9	2.2	0	0
Tomato:								
Raw	1 cup	35	.4	1.6	7.8	3	204	32
Tomato juice	1 cup	42	.1	1.9	10.3	1.7	136	45
Tomato paste	1 cup	220	2.3	10	49	6	647	111
Tomato sauce	1 cup	74	.4	3.2	17.6	3	240	32
Turnips, cooked	1/2 cup	14	0	.6	3.8	1.4	0	9
Vegetable juice	1 cup	46	.2	1.5	11	1.5	283	67
Vegetables, mixed	1 cup	107	.3	5.2	23.8	7.5	779	6
Water chestnuts	1/2 cup	35	0	.6	8.7	.6	0	.9

Index of Tables and Charts

The Vicious Cycle 27
Table 2.1 - Healthful Food Choices 40
Table 3.1 - Glycemic Index 58
Fluid and Electrolyte Replacement Guidline 72
Fat Conversion Guidelines 81
Table 5.1 - Heart Health Numbers 95
Table 5.2 - Fat Content of Condiments 106
Table 5.3 - Fat Content of Snack Foods...... 107
Table 5.4 - Daily Supplement Guide............ 117
Table 6.1 - Antioxidant Sources 132
Table 6.2 - High Fiber Foods........................ 136
Fast Food Tables 165
Smart Food Tables.. 176
Food Value Tables 225

NOTES

Chapter 1

1. "In Search of Longevity,"*East West,* Dec 1989, p.42.
2. "Toward a New Image of Aging," *Prevention*, June 1990, vol. 42, p.103.

Chapter 2

1. Vernon R. Young and Peter L. Pellett, "Protein Intake and Requirements with Reference to Diet and Health," *American Journal of Clinical Nutrition* 45: 1323-1343, 1987.
2. Clive M. McCay, et al., "The Life Span of Rats on a Restricted Diet," *Journal of Nutrition* 18: 1-25, 1939.
3. Clive M. McCay, "Effect of Restricted Feeding Upon Aging and Chronic Diseases in Rats and Dogs," *American Journal of Public Health* 37: 521, 1947.
4. Ronda C. Bell, et al., "NK Cell Activity and Dietary Protein Intake in an Aflatoxin B1(AF)-Induced Tumor Model," *FASEB Journal* (Federation of American Societies for Experimental Biology), Abstract No. 4511, 1990.
5. B. Scott Appleton and T. Colin Campbell, "Inhibition of Aflatoxin-Initiated Preneoplastic Liver Lesions by Low Dietary Protein," *Nutrition and Cancer* 3: 200-206, 1982.
6. Arthur C. Guyton, *Physiology of the Body* (Philadelphia: W.B. Saunders, 1964).

Chapter 3

1. Richard A. Stein, et al., *Consumer Summary,* (Reliance Medical Information, Inc.).
2. *Muscle and Fitness*, Dec 1991, p. 53.
3. Whitney, Caltaldo, Rolfes, *Understanding Normal and Clinical Nutrition,* 1987, p. 80.
4. *Muscle and Fitness*, Dec 1991, p. 130.
5. Whitney, Cataldo, Rolfes, *Understanding Normal and Clinical Nutrition,* 1987, p. 210.
6. Dr. Robert Haas, *Eat to Win* (New York: Rawson Associates, 1983), p.20.
7. Ibid., p. 75.
8. Ibid., p. 77.
9. Ibid., pp. 78-79.

Chapter 5

1. W.B. Kannel and T.J. Thom, *Incidence,Prevalence, and Mortaliy of Cardiovascular diseases in the Heart,* 6th ed., ed. J.W. Hurst (New York: McGraw Hill, 1986), pp. 557-565.
2. Centers for Disease Control, "Years of Life Lost From Cardiovascular Disease," *Journal of the American Medical Association,* 256 : 2794, 1986.
3. *Science News,* 2 Dec 1989, p. 367.
4. *Ibid.*
5. *Ibid.*
6. M.S. Brown and J.S. Goldstein, "Lowering Plasma Cholesterol by Raising LDL Receptors," *New England Journal of Medicine*, 305 : 515-517, 1981.
7. "Weight Down, Cholesterol Up?" *In Health,* Sept/Oct 1991, vol. 5 , No. 5, p. 10.
8. *New England Journal of Medicine,* 16 Aug 1990.
9. Bobbie Hasselbring, *"Reversing Atherosclerosis," HeartCorps*, Dec 1989, vol. 2, p. 59.
10. *Ibid.*
11. *Tufts University Diet and Nutrition Letter,* Sept

1990.
12. *Longevity,* Jan 1991.
13. *Tufts University Diet and Nutrition Letter,* Sept 1990.
14. E. Whitney, C.Cataldo, and S. Rolfes, *Understanding Normal and Clinical Nutrition,* (St. Paul: West Publishing Co., 1987).
15. *New England Journal of Medicine,* 17 Aug 1989, vol. 321, p. 436.
16. *Medicine and Science in Sports and Exercise,* June 1989.
17. *Prevention,* April 1990, vol. 42, p. 12.
18. John Mitchell, "World Conference on Antioxidants Shows Many Preventive Functions," *Health News and Review,* May/June 1990.
19. *Men's Health Newsletter,* May 1991.
20. *Atherosclerosis,* June 1990.
21. *Tufts University Diet and Nutrition Letter,* April 1991.
22. Dr. Julian Whitacker, *Health and Healing,* May 1992, vol. 2, No. 5.
23. Bobbie Hasselbring, "Reversing Atherosclerosis," *HeartCorps,* Dec 1989, p. 59.
24. Dean Ornish, M.D., *Dr. Dean Ornish's Program for Reversing Heart Disease,* 1990, p. 24.

Chapter 6

1. American Cancer Society, *1986 Cancer Facts and Figures,* (New York: American Cancer Society, 1986), p. 3.
2. *Science News,* 18 Feb 1989, p. 102.
3. *Ibid.*
4. *Cancer Research,* 15 August 1990.
5. *Ibid.*
6. *Science News,* 10 Nov 1990.
7. *Health News and Review,* May 1990, vol. 8, p. 1

(2), No. 3.
8. *Ibid.*
9. *Ibid.*
10. *Ibid.*
11. *Ibid.*
12. *University of California at Berkeley Wellness Letter,* Dec 1989.
13. *Ibid.*
14. E. Whitney, C. Cataldo, and S. Rolfes, *Understanding Normal and Clinical Nutrition,* (West Publishing Co.).
15. *American Journal of Epidemiology,* vol. 130, No. 3, 1989.
16. *Medicine and Science in Sports and Exercise,* June 1989.
17. *International Journal of Sports Medicine,* vol. 10, No. 2, 1989.
18. *Nutrition Action Healthletter,* April 1991, p. 5.
19. *bid.*
20. *In Health,* Sept 1991, p. 60.

Chapter 7

1. Dr. Kenneth H. Cooper, *Preventing Osteoporosis,* 1989, p. 7.
2. *New England Journal of Medicine,* 26 June 1986.
3. *Ibid.*
4. *Tufts University Diet and Nutrition Letter,* Sept 1990.
5. *Ibid.*
6. *Total Health,* June 1990, p. 25.
7. *Ibid.*
8. *Ibid.*
9. *American Journal of Epidemiology,* vol. 130, No. 3, 1989.
10. Frederick S. Kaplan, M.D., *Osteoporosis: Pathophysiology and Prevention*, Clinical Sympsia,

CIBA-GEIGY Corp, vol. 39, No. 1, 1987, p. 13.

Chapter 8

1. *Morbidity and Mortality Weekly Report*, 16 Nov 1990, vol. 39, p. 809.
2. "36 Ways to Control Diabetes," *Prevention Magazine,* Sept 1990, vol. 42, p. 62.
3. Whitney, Cataldo, Rolfes, *Understanding Normal and Clinical Nutritition,* 1987, p. 760.
4. Ibid.
5. J.K. Davison, *Non-Insulin-Dependent Diabetes Mellitus*, Clinical Diabetes Mellitus (New York: Thieme, 1986), pp. 11-25.
6. Ibid.
7. *The New England Journal of Medicine,* 25 Jan 1990, vol. 322, p. 262.
8. *Vegetarian Times,* Sept 1990, p. 8.
9. *The New England Journal of Medicine*, 26 June 1986.

BIBLIOGRAPHY

American Cancer Society. *1986 Cancer Facts and Figures.* New York: American Cancer Society, 1986.

American Journal of Epidemiology. vol. 130, No. 3. 1989

Appleton, Scott B. and Campbell, T. Collin. "Inhibition of Aflatoxin-Initiated Preneoplastic Liver Lesions by Low Dietary Protein." *Nutrition and Cancer*, 1982.

Atherosclerosis, June 1990.

Bell, Ronda C. et al. "NK Cell Activity and Dietary Protein Intake in an Aflatoxin B1(AF)-Induced Tumor Model." *FASEB Journal* (Federation of American Societies for Experimental Biology), Abstract No. 4511, 1990.

Brown, M.S., and Godlstein, J.S. "Lowering Plasma Cholesterol by Raising LDL Receptors." *New England Journal of Medicine*, 305 : 1981.

Cancer Research, 15 August 1990.

Centers for Disease Control. "Years of Life Lost From Cardiovascular Disease." *Journal of the American Medical Association*, 256: 2794.

Cooper, Kenneth H.M.D. *Preventing Osteoporosis*, 1989.

Davison, J.K. Non-Insulin-Dependent Diabetes Mellitus, *Clinical Diabetes Mellitus.* New York: Thieme, 1986.

Guyton, Arthur C. *Physiology of the Body.* Philadelphia: W.B. Saunders, 1964.

Haas, Robert M.D. *Eat to Win.* New York: Rawson Associates, 1983.

Hasselbring, Bobbie. "Reversing Atherosclerosis."

Heartcorps, Dec 1989, vol. 2.
Health News and Review, May 1990, vol. 8.
In Health, September 1991.
International Journal of Sports Medicine, vol. 10, No. 2, 1989.
"In Search of Longevity." *East West*, Dec 1989.
Kannel, W.B., and Thom, T.J. *Incidence, Prevalence, and Mortality of Cardiovascular diseases in the Heart,* 6th ed., ed. J.W. Hurst. New York: McGraw-Hill, 1986.
Kaplan, Frederick S. M.D. *Osteoporosis: Pathophysiology and Prevention*, Clinical Sympsia, CIBA-GEIGY Corp, vol. 39, No. 1, 1987.
Longevity, January 1991.
McCay, Clive M. "Effect of Restricted Feeding Upon Aging and Chronic Diseases in Rats and Dogs," *American Journal of Public Health* 37: 521, 1947.
McCay, Clive M., et al. "The Life Span of Rats on a Restricted Diet," *Journal of Nutrition* 18: 1-25, 1939. *Medicine and Science in sports and Exercise,* June 1989.
Men's Health Newsletter, May 1991.
Morbidity and Mortality Weekly Report, 16 Nov 1990.
Mitchel, John. "World Conference on Antioxidants Shows Many Preventive Functions," *Health News and Review,* May/June 1990.
Muscle and Fitness, December 1991.
New England Journal of Medicine, 26 June 1986.
New England Journal of Medicine, 25 January 1986.
New England Journal of Medicine, 16 August 1990.
New England Journal of Medicine, 17 August 1989.
Nutrition Action Healthletter, April 1991.
Ornish, Dean M.D. *Dr. Dean Ornish's Program for Reversing Heart Disease*. 1990.
Prevention, April 1990, vol. 42.
Science News, 18 February 1989.

Science News, 2 December 1989.
Science News, 10 November 1990.
Stein, Richard A. et al. Consumer Summary. *Reliance Medical Information, Inc.*
Total Health, June 1990.
"Toward a New Image of Aging." *Prevention*, vol. 42, June 1990.
Tufts University Diet and Nutrition Letter, September 1990.
Tufts University Diet and Nutrition Letter, April 1991.
University of California at Berkeley Wellness Letter, December 1989.
Vegetarian Times, September 1990.
"36 Ways to Control Diabetes." *Prevention,* September 1990, vol. 42.
"Weight Down, Cholesterol Up?" *In Health*, vol. 5, Sept/Oct 1991.
Whitacker, Julian M.D. *Health and Healing*, May 1992.
Whitney, E., Cataldo, C., and Rolfes, S. *Understanding Normal and Clinical Nutrition.* St. Paul: West Publishing Co., 1987.
Young, Vernon R., and Pellet, Peter L. "Protein Intake and Requirements with Reference to Diet and Health."
American Journal of Clinical Nutrition 45: 1323-1343, 1987.